OTHER FAST FACTS BOOKS

Fast Facts About PTSD: A Guide for Nurses and Other Health Care Professionals (*Adams*)

Fast Facts for the NEW NURSE PRACTITIONER: What You Really Need to Know in a Nutshell, Second Edition (*Aktan*)

Fast Facts for the ER NURSE: Emergency Department Orientation in a Nutshell, Third Edition (*Buettner*)

Fast Facts for the ADULT-GERONTOLOGY ACUTE CARE NURSE PRACTITIONER (*Carpenter*)

Fast Facts About GI AND LIVER DISEASES FOR NURSES: What APRNs Need to Know in a Nutshell (*Chaney*)

Fast Facts for the MEDICAL–SURGICAL NURSE: Clinical Orientation in a Nutshell (*Ciocco*)

Fast Facts on COMBATING NURSE BULLYING, INCIVILITY, AND WORKPLACE VIOLENCE: What Nurses Need to Know in a Nutshell (*Ciocco*)

Fast Facts for the NURSE PRECEPTOR: Keys to Providing a Successful Preceptorship in a Nutshell (*Ciocco*)

Fast Facts for the OPERATING ROOM NURSE: An Orientation and Care Guide, Second Edition (*Criscitelli*)

Fast Facts for the ANTEPARTUM AND POSTPARTUM NURSE: A Nursing Orientation and Care Guide in a Nutshell (*Davidson*)

Fast Facts for the NEONATAL NURSE: A Nursing Orientation and Care Guide in a Nutshell (*Davidson*)

Fast Facts Workbook for CARDIAC DYSRHYTHMIAS AND 12-LEAD EKGs (*Desmarais*)

Fast Facts About PRESSURE ULCER CARE FOR NURSES: How to Prevent, Detect, and Resolve Them in a Nutshell (*Dziedzic*)

Fast Facts for the GERONTOLOGY NURSE: A Nursing Care Guide in a Nutshell (*Eliopoulos*)

Fast Facts for the LONG-TERM CARE NURSE: What Nursing Home and Assisted Living Nurses Need to Know in a Nutshell (*Eliopoulos*)

Fast Facts for the CLINICAL NURSE MANAGER: Managing a Changing Workplace in a Nutshell, Second Edition (*Fry*)

Fast Facts for EVIDENCE-BASED PRACTICE IN NURSING: Third Edition (*Godshall*)

Fast Facts for Nurses About HOME INFUSION THERAPY: The Expert's Best Practice Guide in a Nutshell (*Gorski*)

Fast Facts About NURSING AND THE LAW: Law for Nurses in a Nutshell (*Grant, Ballard*)

Fast Facts for the L&D NURSE: Labor & Delivery Orientation in a Nutshell, Second Edition (*Groll*)

Fast Facts for the RADIOLOGY NURSE: An Orientation and Nursing Care Guide in a Nutshell (*Grossman*)

Fast Facts in HEALTH INFORMATICS FOR NURSES (*Hardy*)

Fast Facts on ADOLESCENT HEALTH FOR NURSING AND HEALTH PROFESSIONALS: A Care Guide in a Nutshell (*Herrman*)

Fast Facts for the CRITICAL CARE NURSE, Second Edition (*Hewett*)

Fast Facts for the FAITH COMMUNITY NURSE: Implementing FCN/Parish Nursing in a Nutshell (*Hickman*)

Fast Facts for the CARDIAC SURGERY NURSE: Caring for Cardiac Surgery Patients, Third Edition (*Hodge*)

Fast Facts About the NURSING PROFESSION: Historical Perspectives in a Nutshell (*Hunt*)

Fast Facts for the NURSE PSYCHOTHERAPIST: The Process of Becoming (*Jones, Tusaie*)

Fast Facts for the CLINICAL NURSING INSTRUCTOR: Clinical Teaching in a Nutshell, Third Edition (*Kan, Stabler-Haas*)

Fast Facts for the WOUND CARE NURSE: Practical Wound Management in a Nutshell (*Kifer*)

Fast Facts About EKGs FOR NURSES: The Rules of Identifying EKGs in a Nutshell (*Landrum*)

Fast Facts for the TRAVEL NURSE: Travel Nursing in a Nutshell (*Landrum*)

Fast Facts for the SCHOOL NURSE: What You Need to Know, Third Edition (*Loschiavo*)

Fast Facts to LOVING YOUR RESEARCH PROJECT: A Stress-Free Guide for Novice Researchers in Nursing and Healthcare (*Marshall*)

Fast Facts for MANAGING PATIENTS WITH A PSYCHIATRIC DISORDER: What RNs, NPs, and New Psych Nurses Need to Know (*Marshall*)

Fast Facts About SUBSTANCE USE DISORDERS: What Every Nurse, APRN, and PA Needs to Know (*Marshall, Spencer*)

Fast Facts About CURRICULUM DEVELOPMENT IN NURSING: How to Develop and Evaluate Educational Programs in a Nutshell, Second Edition (*McCoy, Anema*)

Fast Facts for the CATH LAB NURSE (*McCulloch*)

Fast Facts About NEUROCRITICAL CARE: A Quick Reference for the Advanced Practice Provider (*McLaughlin*)

Fast Facts for DNP ROLE DEVELOPMENT: A Career Navigation Guide (*Menonna-Quinn, Tortorella Genova*)

Fast Facts for DEMENTIA CARE: What Nurses Need to Know in a Nutshell (*Miller*)

Fast Facts for HEALTH PROMOTION IN NURSING: Promoting Wellness in a Nutshell (*Miller*)

Fast Facts for STROKE CARE NURSING: An Expert Care Guide, Second Edition (*Morrison*)

Fast Facts for the MEDICAL OFFICE NURSE: What You Really Need to Know in a Nutshell (*Richmeier*)

Fast Facts for the PEDIATRIC NURSE: An Orientation Guide in a Nutshell (*Rupert, Young*)

Fast Facts About FORENSIC NURSING: What You Need to Know (*Scannell*)

Fast Facts About the GYNECOLOGICAL EXAM: A Professional Guide for NPs, PAs, and Midwives, Second Edition (*Secor, Fantasia*)

Fast Facts About MEDICAL CANNABIS AND OPIOIDS: Minimizing Opioid Use Through Cannabis (*Smith, Smith*)

Fast Facts for the STUDENT NURSE: Nursing Student Success in a Nutshell (*Stabler-Haas*)

Fast Facts About RELIGION FOR NURSES: Implications for Patient Care (*Taylor*)

Fast Facts for CAREER SUCCESS IN NURSING: Making the Most of Mentoring in a Nutshell (*Vance*)

Fast Facts for the TRIAGE NURSE: An Orientation and Care Guide, Second Edition (*Visser, Montejano*)

Fast Facts for DEVELOPING A NURSING ACADEMIC PORTFOLIO: What You Really Need to Know in a Nutshell (*Wittmann-Price*)

Fast Facts for the HOSPICE NURSE: A Concise Guide to End-of-Life Care (*Wright*)

Fast Facts for the CLASSROOM NURSING INSTRUCTOR: Classroom Teaching in a Nutshell (*Yoder-Wise, Kowalski*)

Forthcoming FAST FACTS Books

Fast Facts for NURSE PRACTITIONERS: Current Practice Essentials for the Clinical Subspecialties (*Aktan*)

Fast Facts for the ER NURSE: Guide to a Successful Emergency Department Orientation, Fourth Edition (*Buettner*)

Fast Facts for WRITING THE DNP PROJECT: Effective Structure, Content, and Presentation (*Christenbery*)

Fast Facts for the NURSE PRECEPTOR: Keys to Providing a Successful Preceptorship, Second Edition (*Ciocco*)

Fast Facts for the NEONATAL NURSE: Care Essentials for Normal and High-Risk Neonates, Second Edition (*Davidson*)

Fast Facts About NEUROPATHIC PAIN: What Advanced Practice Nurses and Physician Assistants Need to Know (*Davies*)

Fast Facts about DIVERSITY, EQUITY, AND INCLUSION (*Davis*)

Fast Facts for the Radiology Nurse: An Orientation and Nursing Care Guide, Second Edition (*Grossman*)

Fast Facts for CREATING A SUCCESSFUL TELEHEALTH SERVICE: A How-to Guide for Nurse Practitioners (*Heidesch*)

Fast Facts for PATIENT SAFETY IN NURSING (*Hunt*)

Fast Facts for DEMENTIA CARE: What Nurses Need to Know, Second Edition (*Miller*)

Fast Facts for NURSE ANESTHESIA (*Moore, Hickman*)

Fast Facts for MAKING THE MOST OF YOUR CAREER IN NURSING (*Redulla*)

Fast Facts for PEDIATRIC PRIMARY CARE: A Guide for Nurse Practitioners and Physician Assistants (*Ruggiero*)

Fast Facts About SEXUALLY TRANSMITTED INFECTIONS (STIs): A Nurse's Guide to Expert Patient Care (*Scannell*)

Fast Facts About LGBTQ CARE FOR NURSES (*Traister*)

Fast Facts for the CLINICAL NURSE LEADER (*Wilcox, Deerhake*)

Fast Facts About COMPETENCY-BASED EDUCATION IN NURSING: How to Teach Competency Mastery (*Wittmann-Price, Gittings*)

Fast Facts for the HOSPICE NURSE: A Concise Guide to End-of-Life Care, Second Edition (*Wright*)

Visit www.springerpub.com to order.

FAST FACTS About
MEDICAL CANNABIS AND OPIOIDS

Gregory L. Smith, MD, MPH, earned his medical degree from Rush Medical School in Chicago and a master's of public health from Harvard University. He completed residency training in preventive medicine at Walter Reed Army Medical Center. He is a former major in the U.S. Army and has had extensive experience and education in the field of cannabinoid medications.

His previous book, *Medical Cannabis: Basic Science and Clinical Applications,* is a scientifically based textbook directed at educating medical students and medical professionals on the science and applications of cannabinoid medications. He has also written *CBD: What You Need to Know,* designed to empower the average patient and caregiver with the effects of cannabidiol (CBD).

Dr. Smith consults as a scientific and medical adviser on cannabis and cannabinoid therapeutics with over a dozen companies in four countries.

Kevin F. Smith, MD, MPH, completed his medical degree and then went on to receive a master's of public health from Yale University while completing residency in occupational and preventive medicine at both Yale and the University of Iowa.

As a board-certified physician, Dr. Smith's 30-odd years' experience has seen his broad skillset coalesce into sought-after expertise. He has provided leadership as the medical director and the director of medical operations (DMO) for multiple healthcare systems, including a large healthcare system in Northwest Ohio ranked as a top 50 hospital system in the United States.

While in the U.S. Army Reserve Medical Corps, Dr. Kevin F. Smith reached the status of lieutenant colonel. He has been deployed several times, in the capacity of field surgeon and preventive medicine physician.

Expert Consultant

Nikki Wright, MBA, holds an MBA from Portland State University and a BSc from Humboldt State University. She is the chief operations officer at Medical Marijuana 411 and has spearheaded the monumental task of working with doctors and cannabinoid experts to create continuing medical education (CME) activities for physicians, nurses, and pharmacists. Recent CME activities include Medical Marijuana Continuing Medical Education and FDA-Approved Cannabinoid Medications.

FAST FACTS About
MEDICAL CANNABIS AND OPIOIDS

Minimizing Opioid Use Through Cannabis

Gregory L. Smith, MD, MPH
Kevin F. Smith, MD, MPH

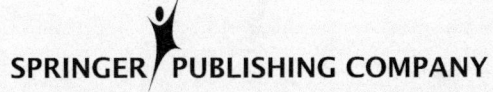

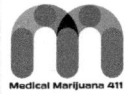

Copyright © 2021 Springer Publishing Company, LLC

All rights reserved.

No part of this publication may be reproduced, stored in a retrieval system, or transmitted in any form or by any means, electronic, mechanical, photocopying, recording, or otherwise, without the prior permission of Springer Publishing Company, LLC, or authorization through payment of the appropriate fees to the Copyright Clearance Center, Inc., 222 Rosewood Drive, Danvers, MA 01923, 978-750-8400, fax 978-646-8600, info@copyright.com or on the Web at www.copyright.com.

Springer Publishing Company, LLC
11 West 42nd Street, New York, NY 10036
www.springerpub.com
connect.springerpub.com/

Acquisitions Editor: Rachel Landes
Compositor: Amnet Systems
Photo credits: Joshua Rainey/123 RF (Figure 9.1); Mitch M./Shutterstock (Figure 9.2); Dalyn/Adobe Stock Photo (Figure 9.3); Capjah/Shutterstock (Figure 9.4).

ISBN: 978-0-8261-4299-3
ebook ISBN: 978-0-8261-4312-9
DOI: 10.1891/9780826143129

20 21 22 23 24 / 5 4 3 2 1

Medicine is an ever-changing science. Research and clinical experience are continually expanding our knowledge, in particular our understanding of proper treatment and drug therapy. The authors, editors, and publisher have made every effort to ensure that all information in this book is in accordance with the state of knowledge at the time of production of the book. Nevertheless, the authors, editors, and publisher are not responsible for any errors or omissions or for any consequence from application of the information in this book and make no warranty, expressed or implied, with respect to the content of this publication. Every reader should examine carefully the package inserts accompanying each drug and should carefully check whether the dosage schedules therein or the contraindications stated by the manufacturer differ from the statements made in this book. Such examination is particularly important with drugs that are either rarely used or have been newly released on the market.

Library of Congress Cataloging-in-Publication Data
Names: Smith, Gregory L., author. | Smith, Kevin (Kevin F.), author.
Title: Fast facts about medical cannabis and opioids : minimizing opioid
  use through cannabis / Gregory Smith, Kevin Smith.
Other titles: Fast facts (Springer Publishing Company)
Description: New York, NY : Springer Publishing Company, LLC, [2021] |
  Series: Fast facts | Includes bibliographical references and index.
Identifiers: LCCN 2019052520 (print) | LCCN 2019052521 (ebook) | ISBN
  9780826142993 (paperback) | ISBN 9780826143129 (ebook)
Subjects: MESH: Chronic Pain—drug therapy | Pain Management |
  Cannabinoids—therapeutic use | Medical Marijuana—therapeutic use |
  Analgesics, Opioid—adverse effects | Opioid-Related
  Disorders—prevention & control | Nurses Instruction
Classification: LCC RM666.C266 (print) | LCC RM666.C266 (ebook) | NLM WL
  704.6 | DDC 615.3/23648—dc23
LC record available at https://lccn.loc.gov/2019052520
LC ebook record available at https://lccn.loc.gov/2019052521

Contact us to receive discount rates on bulk purchases.
We can also customize our books to meet your needs.
For more information please contact: sales@springerpub.com

Publisher's Note: New and used products purchased from third-party sellers are not guaranteed for quality, authenticity, or access to any included digital components.

Printed in the United States of America.

This book is dedicated to Jack, Mark, and Frank. Thank you for your extraordinary mentorship and continuous encouragement throughout this process. Your unwavering belief in the work we are doing and the potential benefits to patients keeps us moving forward every day.

Contents

Preface — xi
Acknowledgments — xiii

Part I THE OPIOID EPIDEMIC

1. Chronic Pain and Opioids — 3
2. Current Costs of the Opioid Epidemic — 13
3. Opioid Use Disorder — 23

Part II OVERVIEW OF CANNABIS

4. History and Legality of Cannabis — 39
5. Overview of the Endocannabinoid System — 55

Part III CANNABINOIDS

6. Cannabinoids and Terpenes — 73
7. Synthetic Cannabinoid Pharmaceuticals — 87
8. Isolate Cannabinoid Pharmaceuticals — 95

Part IV MEDICAL MARIJUANA

9. Medical Marijuana and Bioavailability — 107
10. Side Effects of Cannabis Use — 125

Part V CHRONIC PAIN MANAGEMENT

11. Causes of Chronic Pain	139
12. Treating Chronic Pain With Opioids	151
13. Treating Chronic Pain With Cannabinoids	165

Part VI CANNABINOIDS AND THE OPIOID CRISIS

14. Cannabinoid and Opioid Interactions	179
15. Cannabis as an Adjunct to Opioids	191
16. Opioid Sparing With Cannabinoids	199

Appendix A. Centers for Disease Control and Prevention Guideline for Prescribing Opioids for Chronic Pain — *213*

Appendix B. National Institutes of Drug Abuse Quick Screen and NIDA-Modified ASSIST Screenings for Opioid Use Disorder — *215*

Appendix C. Centers for Disease Control and Prevention Calculating Total Daily Dose of Opioids for Safer Dosage — *227*

Index — *229*

Preface

Welcome to *Fast Facts About Medical Cannabis and Opioids: Minimizing Opioid Use Through Cannabis*. This book is an overview about how cannabinoids can play an integral part in a patient's pain management treatment plan. It is a resource for anyone working with patients experiencing chronic noncancer-related pain, including physician assistants, nurse practitioners, clinical nurse specialists, and bedside nurses.

We wrote this book to be able to give you an unbiased look into how cannabis has helped with pain management for thousands of years and what is driving the resurgence in patient use. The opioid crisis has reached epidemic proportions with 130 people dying daily from complications of opioid use. Cannabis may be a way to combat the crisis, help relieve pain, and reverse opioid addiction rates.

Right now patients are self-medicating throughout the country with no supervision from their medical providers. It is estimated there are 3.5 million patients in the United States who are using medical marijuana to treat a myriad of ailments. This book is intended to be a tool for you to answer basic questions about medical cannabis and how it works in the body and gives an overview of the endocannabinoid system. Our goal at Medical Marijuana 411 is to give you the tools to provide unbiased, accurate information that you can share with your patients. Cannabis has many benefits being discovered daily, but it is also a drug, not a miracle cure. We hope that this publication helps you have open, honest conversations with your patients to give them the best care experience possible.

Nikki Wright
Cofounder
Medical Marijuana 411

Acknowledgments

To Chris Nazarenus, our leader and visionary, thank you for your unwavering belief in providing world-class educational material that has inspired us to create outstanding content. You have taught us not only to produce the best products but also to foster a platform that ultimately improves a patient's quality of life. Without you none of this would be possible!

To our advisers and mentors who have been with us every step of the way. You have all had a hand in helping us move past roadblocks and achieve new goals we never thought possible. Thank you, Mark Mersman, for bringing us together as a powerhouse team of experts and helping us navigate the continuing medical education (CME) hurdles when we thought success was out of reach. Thank you, Dr. Jack Cox, for teaching us that information is vital to the medical community even when it may be viewed as controversial. Also, thank you for completing multiple reviews during nights, weekends, and even when you were moving from state to state. Thank you, Frank Costanzo, for guiding us through the publishing world and helping us dive into a new medium. This whole crazy experience has given us a new respect for publishing. And a special thanks to Greg Tracy for always steering us in the right direction throughout this entire endeavor.

To our amazing editors, Elizabeth Nieginski and Rachel Landes, thank you for your positivity and always being available to answer questions. On more than a few occasions, you responded to emails well into the night. Your expertise and guidance were invaluable throughout the process. We couldn't have done it without you!

Many thanks to Rick Beets, Michelle Clement, and Lane Trachy for your extraordinary technical support, research assistance, and overall help moving projects forward. We cannot express enough how lucky we are to have you support us in all our endeavors to bring cannabis education to the world.

The Opioid Epidemic

1

Chronic Pain and Opioids

The opioid crisis in America is worsening daily with addiction rates and the associated costs soaring. This chapter discusses the issues around chronic pain, opioid use, and the resulting epidemic of opioid dependency and abuse.

In this chapter, you will learn how to:

- Define pain and categories of pain.
- Review issues related to the chronic pain epidemic.
- Compare clinical studies related to opioid use.
- List issues associated with the opioid epidemic.

CHRONIC PAIN

Pain is a widespread phenomenon that affects over 100 million Americans—more than diabetes, heart disease, and cancer combined. An estimated 20% of American adults (approximately 42 million people) report that pain or physical discomfort disrupts their sleep a few nights a week or more. The World Health Organization (WHO) recognizes pain as a global public health concern.

Definition of Pain

Pain is a warning signal that the body is experiencing imminent or actual damage. The International Association for the Study of Pain defines pain as, "An unpleasant sensory and emotional experience arising from actual or potential tissue damage or described in terms of such damage" (IASP, 1994, pp. 209–214).

Pain is a critical function for protection; it helps to prevent damage and helps the body return to normal functioning, but it can also be experienced occasionally in the absence of tissue damage or after the original injury has healed.

Fast Facts

Pain is not only a sensory experience, but it also impacts patients emotionally.

Overview of Pain

- Pain is the most common reason that a person seeks medical care.
- Reports of pain levels by patients are influenced by their tolerance of pain.
- Pain has sensory and emotional components.

Fast Facts

Pain can be a chronic disease and a barrier to cancer treatment; it can occur alongside other diseases and conditions.

Recent Issues in Pain

- Pain affects more Americans than diabetes, heart disease, and cancer combined.
- Chronic pain is the most common cause of long-term disability.
- The Centers for Disease Control and Prevention (CDC, 2019) has provided *Guidelines for Prescribing Opioids for Chronic Pain* (see Appendix A) given that an estimated 11% of adults experience daily pain.

Fast Facts

Chronic and recurrent pain should be viewed as a disease in its own right, which poses a significant health burden.

CHRONIC PAIN EPIDEMIC

Chronic pain has reached epidemic proportions in the past decade, with an estimated 80 million current chronic pain sufferers in the United States. There has been concomitant exponential growth in the use of prescription opioids for chronic pain. Currently, the United States consumes 80% of the world's supply of prescription opioids. A significant proportion of chronic pain patients are also being treated with addictive benzodiazepines, and 33% of prescription opioid overdose cases also involved taking a benzodiazepine.

Much of this increase in opioid use has been due to:

- Relaxed prescription guidelines for nonmalignant pain
- Aggressive pharmaceutical marketing campaigns even though there is little research to support long-term use of opioids for chronic nonmalignant pain

See Box 1.1 for the associated consequences of the opioid epidemic.

Fast Facts

Chronic pain involves the interaction of physical, psychological, and social factors.

BOX 1.1 ASSOCIATED CONSEQUENCES OF THE OPIOID EPIDEMIC

- There has been a fourfold increase in the number of deaths from prescription opioids between 1999 and 2011
- The CDC estimates that 130 people a day die from prescription opioid overdose and a total of 33,000 unintentional deaths occurred in 2015
- There are over 700,000 opioid-related hospitalizations annually
  - As many as 60% of these overdose deaths involved patients with prescribed opioids, who were not using the drugs illicitly
- Prolonged periods of abstinence from opioids, due to lack of access or other issues, may lead to unexpected overdose when the patient resumes the previous tolerated dose
- There has been a dramatic increase in ED visits for unintentional overdoses of opioids by young children and intentional use of family member's opioids by adolescents

> **Fast Facts**
>
> *Unintentional opioid overdoses are associated with preventable factors: stopping the concomitant use of benzodiazepine or advising patients not to resume the use of opioids at previously tolerated elevated doses.*

OPIOID USE

The epidemic of opioid prescriptions flies in the face of evidence that opioids are only modestly useful for chronic pain. Moreover, long-term use is often associated with adverse effects and requires the use of other prescription medications to treat them.

Long-Term Effects of Opioids

- Nausea and vomiting
- Abdominal distention and bloating
- Constipation
- Liver damage
- Brain damage due to hypoxia
- Development of tolerance
- Dependence

Recent Study Findings

A recent meta-analysis of 96 randomized clinical trials looked at a total of 26,169 patients with chronic noncancer pain. However, the most frequent observation time was 4 weeks, which inhibited the researchers' ability to identify long-term pain and functioning benefits from opioids.

- Findings showed a small, yet significant, ($p < .05$) improvement of pain and physical functioning compared to placebo.
- Researchers were unable to identify adverse effects and complicating conditions with prolonged opioid use.

Analysis of Veteran's Administration (VA) data has shown that higher doses of opioids for chronic noncancer pain are associated with a much higher risk for opioid-related complications. Another VA study of almost 1 million veterans found that 71% of patients who are started on opioids and maintained on them for at least 90 days will still be taking opioids 3 years later (Figure 1.1).

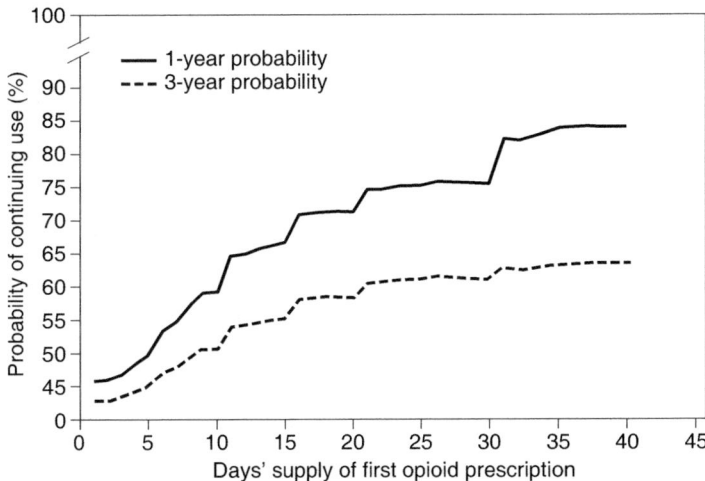

Figure 1.1 One- and 3-year probabilities of continued opioid use among opioid-naive patients, by number of days supply* of the first opioid prescription;United States, 2006–2015.

*Days supply of the first prescription is expressed in days (1–40) in 1-day increments. If a patient had multiple prescriptions on the first day, the prescription with the longest days supply was considered the first prescription.

Source: Shah, A., Hayes, C. J., & Martin, B. C. (2017). Characteristics of initial prescription episodes and likelihood of long-term opioid use—U.S., 2006–2015. *MMWR Morbidity and Mortality Weekly Report, 66*(10), 265–269.

A study comparing opioids with nonopioid medications and pain-related function over 12 months found:

- Opioids were not superior to nonopioid medications for severe chronic back pain or hip or knee osteoarthritis pain.
- Use of nonopioid medications for acute pain could prevent the eventual chronic use of opioids.

Fast Facts

Several studies have found that combining over-the-counter doses of acetaminophen and nonsteroidal anti-inflammatory drugs (NSAIDs) are as effective as opioids for acute pain.

EPIDEMIC OF OPIOID DEPENDENCY AND ABUSE

Chronic pain patients are commonly denied additional prescriptions for opioids due to failed urine drug testing, most often from cannabis obtained illicitly for opioid sparing. Unfortunately, when these opioid-dependent patients suddenly lose their prescription, they may seek out opioids illegally.

Research has shown that, over time, due to lack of access and cost issues, these patients often end up using heroin "off the street," which is increasingly cut with fentanyl or with the exponentially more potent carfentanyl. Fentanyl is 100 times more potent than morphine. See Box 1.2 for information on the consequences of increased heroin use.

BOX 1.2 CONSEQUENCES OF INCREASED HEROIN USE

- Greatly increases the chance of unintended fatal overdose (see also Figure 1.2).
- Twenty-six people die each day for heroin-related overdoses.
  - As many as 80% of these deaths were patients who became addicted to opioids after being prescribed opioids for an injury or surgery.

RESPONSE TO THE OPIOID EPIDEMIC

About 2.1 million persons in the United States live with opioid use disorder (OUD). There has been a public and political outcry as efforts over the past few years have failed to significantly reverse these statistics.

The CDC released a report in 2016 entitled *Prescribing Opioids for Chronic Pain*. This guideline excluded palliative or end-of-life care.

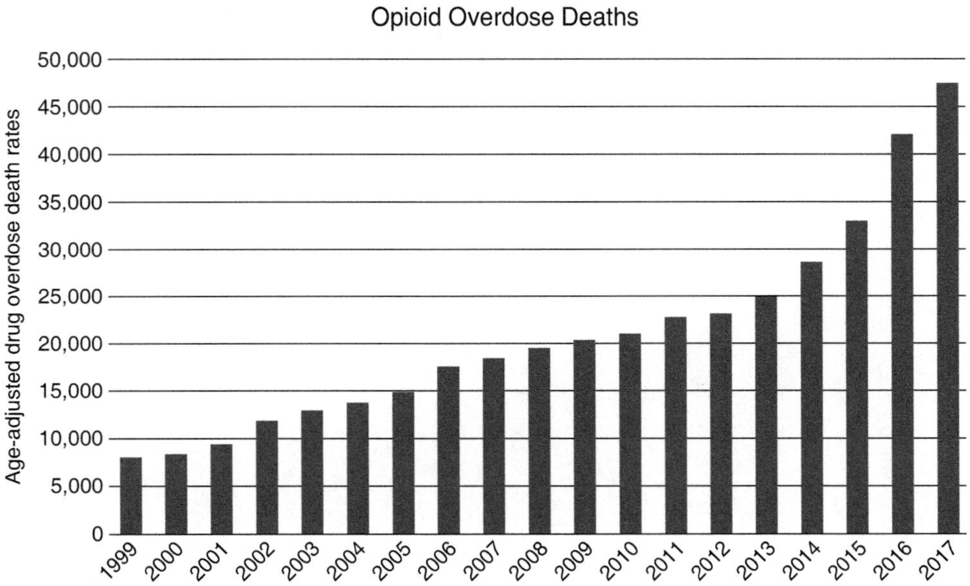

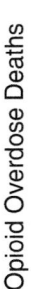

Figure 1.2 National drug overdose deaths involving any opioid, 1999–2017.
Source: CDC WONDER. Retrieved from https://wonder.cdc.gov/mcd.html.

There are several key takeaways:

- In general, do not prescribe opioids as the first-line treatment for chronic pain.
- Avoid concurrent opioid and benzodiazepine use whenever possible.
- Benzodiazepines or sedating muscle relaxants, such as opioids, are respiratory depressants. They work synergistically—opioids at receptors in the medulla oblongata and benzodiazepines and muscle relaxants as CNS depressants.
  - The Food and Drug Administration (FDA) has recently added a black box warning to address this.
- Use of medical cannabis or FDA-approved cannabinoid medications (CMs) as adjunct therapy may be a significant part of the solution.
  - CMs:
    - Have been shown to have efficacy in opioid sparing as an alternative analgesic
    - Can be used for mood elevation
    - Can be used for reducing opioid withdrawal and craving
- Ongoing problems include:
  - Prevention of relapse, which is extremely common
  - As many as 85% of individuals in abstinence-based programs relapse within 12 months

Programs using medication assisted treatment (MAT) with buprenorphine or methadone show somewhat superior long-term results, but they still have high rates of relapse. In addition, the number of buprenorphine-certified providers or methadone programs is significantly limited, especially in rural areas where they are often most needed.

References

Centers for Disease Control and Prevention. (2019). *Guideline for prescribing opioids for chronic pain.* Washington, DC: Centers for Disease Control and Prevention.

IASP. (1994). Part III: Pain terms, a current list with definitions and notes on usage. In H. Merskey & N. Bogduk (Eds.), *Classification of Chronic Pain, Second Edition, IASP Task Force on Taxonomy* (pp. 209–214). Seattle: ISAP Press.

Bibliography

Busse, J. W., Wang, L., Kamaleldin, M., Craigie, S., Riva, J. J., Montoya, L., ... Guyatt, G. H. (2019). Opioids for chronic noncancer pain: A systematic review and meta-analysis. *JAMA, 320*(23), 2448–2460. doi:10.1001/jama.2018.18472

Chang, A. K., Bijur, P. E., Esses, D., Barnaby, D. P., & Baer, J. (2018). Effect of a single dose of oral opioid and nonopioid analgesics on acute extremity pain in the emergency department: A randomized clinical trial. *JAMA, 318*(17), 1661–1667. doi:10.1001/jama.2017.16190

Dowell, D., Haegerich, T. M., & Chou, R. (2016). CDC guideline for prescribing opioids for chronic pain—United States, 2016. *MMWR Recommendations and Reports, 65*(1), 1–49. doi:10.15585/mmwr.rr6501e1

Hedegaard, H., Warner, M., & Miniño, A. M. (2017). Drug overdose deaths in the United States, 1999–2016. *NCHS Data Brief* (294), 1–8.

Institute of Medicine. (2011). *Relieving pain in America: A blueprint for transforming prevention, care, education, and research*. Washington, DC: The National Academies Press.

Krebs, E. E., Gravely, A., Nugent, S., Jensen, A. C., DeRonne, B., Goldsmith, E. S., ... Noorbaloochi, S. (2018). Effect of opioid vs. nonopioid medications on pain-related function in patients with chronic back pain or hip or knee osteoarthritis pain: The SPACE randomized clinical trial. *JAMA, 319*(9), 872–882. doi:10.1001/jama.2018.0899

Morasco, B. J., Duckart, J. P., Carr, T. P., Deyo, R. A., & Dobscha, S. K. (2010). Clinical characteristics of veterans prescribed high doses of opioid medications for chronic non-cancer pain. *Pain, 151*(3), 625–632. doi:10.1016/j.pain.2010.08.002

Morasco, B. J., Krebs, E. E., Adams, M. H., Hyde, S., Zamudio, J., & Dobscha, S. K. (2019). Clinician response to aberrant urine drug test results of patients prescribed opioid therapy for chronic pain. *The Clinical Journal of Pain, 35*(1), 1–6. doi:10.1097/AJP.0000000000000652

National Institutes of Health. (2010). *Pain management fact sheet*. Retrieved from https://report.nih.gov/NIHfactsheets/Pdfs/PainManagement(NINR).pdf

National Sleep Foundation—Sleep Research & Education. (2017). *Sleep foundation.org*. Retrieved from http://www.sleepfoundation.org

Ong, C. K., Seymour, R. A., Lirk, P., & Merry, A. F. (2010). Combining paracetamol (acetaminophen) with nonsteroidal anti-inflammatory drugs: A qualitative systematic review of analgesic efficacy for acute postoperative pain. *Anesthesia and Analgesia, 110*(4), 1170–1179. doi:10.1213/ANE.0b013e3181cf9281

Pain Management Information. (2019). *Definition of pain*. Retrieved from http://pain-management-info.com/definition-of-pain/

Rose, M. E. (2018). Are prescription opioids driving the opioid crisis? Assumptions vs. facts. *Pain Medicine, 19*(4), 793–807. doi:10.1093/pm/pnx048

Rudd, R. A., Seth, P., David, F., & Scholl, L. (2019). Increases in drug and opioid-involved overdose deaths—United States, 2010–2015. *MMWR*

Recommendations and Reports, 65(50–51), 1445–1452. doi:10.15585/mmwr.mm655051e1

Slawson, D. C. (2018). Ibuprofen plus acetaminophen equals opioid plus acetaminophen for acute severe extremity pain. *American Family Physician, 97*(5), 348.

U.S. Food and Drug. (2017). Drug safety and availability—FDA Drug Safety Communication: FDA warns about serious risks and death when combining opioid pain or cough medicines with benzodiazepines; requires its strongest warning. Silver Spring, MD: U.S. Food and Drug Administration.

Wiese, B., & Wilson-Poe, A. R. (2018). Emerging evidence for cannabis' role in opioid use disorder. *Cannabis and Cannabinoid Research, 3*(1), 179–189. doi:10.1089/can.2018.0022

2

Current Costs of the Opioid Epidemic

The costs of the opioid epidemic need to be measured in several different ways to gain a true understanding of the impact. This chapter discusses the cost to patients, the healthcare system, and the economy.

In this chapter, you will learn how to:

- Understand all the direct and indirect financial costs of the opioid epidemic.
- List the various ways that healthcare expenses are impacted by the opioid epidemic.
- List how the impact of the epidemic affects workplace productivity.

ESTIMATING THE COSTS OF OPIOIDS

There are the financial costs, including healthcare expenses and the economic impact of lost productivity. The financial costs also include costs associated with incarceration and for attempts to achieve future harm reduction. Last but not least, there are the unquantifiable costs associated with the huge impact on families, communities, and society in general from the 130 unintentional deaths a day of young people using these drugs.

Fast Facts

In 2017, the high rate of unintentional opioid-related deaths, mostly in younger people, reversed the average life expectancy in the United States for the first time in decades.

We know the cost to society of the opioid epidemic in terms of lives lost. However, to calculate the current economic costs of the epidemic, we need to look at a myriad of direct and indirect costs.

Direct and Indirect Costs

- Healthcare
- Workplace
- Criminal justice
- Society

Earlier estimates seriously underestimated treatment costs. In the 2016 research, 82% of persons with substance abuse disorders did not receive adequate treatment. Over time, the use of more expensive medically assisted treatment (MAT) is expected to significantly increase, along with lifetime use of pharmaceuticals.

In 2013, the Centers for Disease Control and Prevention (CDC) estimated that the total "economic burden" of prescription opioid misuse, dependence, and overdose in the United States alone costs $78.5 billion a year (Exhibit 2.1). These financial resources are not only being used in response to a preventable epidemic, but they are also being used at the expense of programs and healthcare for other important nonpreventable conditions.

The 2013 CDC analysis showed over one third of the expenses, $28.9 billion, was directly related to healthcare and substance abuse treatment. Out-of-pocket expenses to the patient are often barriers to treatment of opioid use disorder (OUD), except for emergency medical services.

However, the proportion of people with OUD who can access long-term drug rehabilitation treatment is expected to significantly increase as these services become more available. The Mental Health Parity and Addiction Equity Act (MHPAEA) passed in 2008 created wider access to rehabilitation services, expanded the use of new opioid treatment medications, and broadened other substance use disorder treatment access initiatives.

Exhibit 2.1

Aggregate Societal Costs of Prescription Opioid Abuse, Dependence, and Fatal Overdose: United States (Millions of 2013 Dollars)

Nonfatal Costs	Aggregate Costs	Percentage of Aggregate Costs
Healthcare		
Private insurance	$14,041	17.90%
Medicare	$2,593*	3.30%
Medicaid	$5,490*	7.00%
Champus/Veterans Affairs	$428*	0.50%
Other	$1,003	1.30%
Uninsured	$2,519	3.20%
Total	**$26,075**	**33.20%**
Substance abuse treatment		
Federal	$721*	0.90%
State and local	$1,823*	2.30%
Private	$276	0.40%
Total	**$2,820**	**3.60%**
Criminal justice		
Police protection	$2,812*	3.60%
Legal and adjudication	$1,288*	1.60%
Correctional facilities	$3,218*	4.10%
Property lost due to crime	$335	0.40%
Total	**$7,654**	**9.70%**
Lost productivity		
Reduced productive time/increased disability	$16,262	20.70%
Production lost for incarcerated individuals	$4,180	5.30%
Total	**$20,441**	**26.00%**
Total	**$56,990**	**72.60%**

(continued)

Exhibit 2.1

Aggregate Societal Costs of Prescription Opioid Abuse, Dependence, and Fatal Overdose: United States (Millions of 2013 Dollars) *(continued)*

Nonfatal Costs	Aggregate Costs	Percentage of Aggregate Costs
Fatal costs		
Lost productivity	$21,429	27.30%
Healthcare	$84	0.10%
Total	**$21,513**	**27.40%**
GRAND TOTAL	**$78,503**	**100.00%**

* Denotes public sector costs.
Source: Reproduced with permission from Florence, C. S., Zhou, C., Luo, F., & Xu, L. (2016). The economic burden of prescription opioid overdose, abuse and dependence in the United States, 2013. *Medical Care, 54*(10), 901–906. doi:10.1097/MLR.0000000000000625.

MEDICALLY ASSISTED THERAPY COSTS

The medical community and state legislatures are gradually adopting the MAT theory of treatment, over detoxification, abstinence, and 12-step programs. The SUPPORT for Patients and Communities Act was signed into law in 2018 and reauthorized funding for the 21st Century Act that put $500 million a year toward the opioid crisis. This Act improved physician access, flexibility, and reimbursement for MAT treatment.

Medications Approved by the Food and Drug Administration for Use in MAT

- Methadone
- Buprenorphine
- Naltrexone

Each drug is subject to numerous regulations, with those applying to methadone being the strictest.

According to MAT, opioid addiction is a chronic brain disease that needs to be treated for a lifetime with opioid antagonist drugs in combination with behavioral therapy. MAT programs are usually conducted for outpatients with a combination of pharmacotherapy with opioid antagonists and/or agonists, and outpatient psychosocial therapy. Many studies have shown that such MAT programs are superior to pharmacotherapy alone, such as with methadone programs, abstinence, or 12-step programs.

Fast Facts

In the first long-term follow-up of patients treated with buprenorphine/naloxone for OUD, 50% reported that they were abstinent from the drugs 18 months after starting the therapy. After 3.5 years, the proportion who reported being abstinent had risen further, to 61%.

Historically, substance abuse rehabilitation has followed the 12-step program, going back to the 1930s. As physician expertise with MAT programs developed over the past few years, programs gradually transitioned from traditional 12-step programs to MAT, with or without a 12-step component. However, as recently as 2015, three fourths of inpatient drug rehabilitation programs did not have MAT.

An analysis of the costs of MAT for OUD used data from large, private, employer-sponsored health plans, and as well Kaiser and Brandeis health plans. The study featured an "ideal treatment protocol for a typical individual with OUD." The services included some cases that required detoxification. The model allowed for 18 physician office visits, 15 psychotherapy visits, and 12 monthly buprenorphine prescription fills per year. The average annual cost was $6,886 per patient in 2014.

Fast Facts

"Presenteeism" is a recently developed concept where the employee is at work and being paid, but is impaired and underproductive due to the cognitive and psychosocial effects of the opioids, addiction, and/or MAT.

UNNECESSARY URINE DRUG TESTING COSTS

While baseline and regular urine drug tests (UDT) are appropriate, testing can be accomplished effectively and inexpensively with a simple six-panel qualitative UDT. A definitive, very extensive series of tests with quantitative measurements of each drug and metabolite is rarely necessary.

> **Fast Facts**
>
> *A qualitative test tells you if a particular substance (analyte) is present in the urine specimen. A quantitative test tells you how much (the quantity) of an analyte is present.*

Unfortunately, the potential for huge profits from "definitive" or quantitative drug testing has led to an exponential increase in the number and frequency of quantitative drug testing both for patients being prescribed opioids or those in drug rehabilitation programs. A typical qualitative UDT at baseline and annually for six drugs of abuse costs about $45. However, a detailed quantitative analysis of dozens of drugs costs as much as $2,500. Some physician offices order this test every visit and make well over a thousand dollars in profit on each test.

UNDERESTIMATED COSTS

In 2017, the Council of Economic Advisors to the Executive Branch of the U.S. government put out an extensive report entitled "The Underestimated Cost of the Opioid Crisis," which estimated that 2.4 million adults had OUD in 2016. They found that previous reports had significantly underestimated the economic cost of the deaths from unintentional opioid overdose. The council estimated the opioid crisis in 2015 cost $504 billion, or 2.8% of the gross domestic product, six times the recent underestimate (see Table 2.1).

Table 2.1

Estimated Costs of the Opioid Crisis in 2015 (2015 $)

Fatality Costs	Nonfatality Costs	Total Costs
$431.7 billion	$72.3 billion	$504 billion

Source: The White House. (2017, November). *Council of Economic Advisers. The underestimated cost of the opioid crisis*. Executive Office of the President. Retrieved from https://www.whitehouse.gov/briefings-statements/cea-report-underestimated-cost-opioid-crisis/.

In changing the estimates, the council found that previously 73% of the cost was attributed to nonfatal consequences, including healthcare costs, criminal justice costs, and lost productivity due to absenteeism, presenteeism, and incarceration. Twenty-seven percent was attributed to the fatality costs consisting of lost potential earnings.

> **Fast Facts**
>
> *The American Society for Addiction Medicine (ASAM) released a 66-page National Practice Guideline for the Use of Medications in the Treatment of Addiction Involving Opioid Use from 2015. It has no mention of the potential use of cannabinoids for OUD.*

The Council used updated calculations for financial impact of the lives being lost, emphasizing that most opioid-related deaths occur at the ages of maximum income earning and in those who are heads of household, namely between 25 and 55 years of age. The Council further identified that in 2014, 24% of the opioid-related overdose deaths were underreported on death certificates. With the new corrected estimate. fatality-related costs were 85% of the total cost.

> **Fast Facts**
>
> *Neonatal abstinence syndrome due to opioid use and misuse during pregnancy is increasing significantly. There was a fivefold increase in the number of neonates born with this condition between 2004 and 2014, when 32,000 babies were diagnosed with this syndrome.*

WORKPLACE AND PRODUCTIVITY COSTS

There are several ways that OUD impacts the workplace and productivity.

- Absenteeism due to health or psychosocial effects
- Absenteeism due to incarceration
- Prolonged hospitalization or death
- Impairment from cognitive and proprioceptive effects
- Increased rates of on-the-job injuries and accidents

A newer phenomenon known as "presenteeism" may have an even bigger economic impact than the $1,685 per employee per year attributed to absenteeism. Presenteeism refers to employees who come to work sick, fatigued, or impaired from prescribed or illicit drugs, alcohol, physical, or psychosocial factors. The cost of absenteeism and presenteeism from opioids was estimated to be $10 billion.

> **Fast Facts**
>
> *"Presenteeism," or working while sick, can cause productivity loss, poor health, exhaustion, and workplace epidemics.*

UNACCOUNTED COSTS

After looking at all the estimated costs and expected changes as the epidemic evolves, costs will go unaccounted for or be seriously underestimated.

Caregiver Burden

Over 2.5 million grandparents are estimated to now act as foster parents of their own grandchildren. Instead of state-structured foster programs, 30% of foster children are now living with relatives. The financial burden on grandparents and close relatives has yet to be estimated. This is known as "caregiver burden."

> **Fast Facts**
>
> *The economic costs of close family members who are impacted by the many, often disastrous, psychosocial effects of having a family member with OUD have yet to be calculated.*

Adverse Effects Treatment

The costs of using long-term nonopioid drugs to treat the severe adverse effects from long-term opioid use such as opioid-induced constipation (OIC), depression, and hypogonadism have not been included in the healthcare models.

> **Fast Facts**
>
> *OIC is a debilitating side effect of opioid therapy, with symptoms persisting for the duration of treatment.*

A retrospective case–control study using commercial and Medicare database evaluated 401 nonelderly and 194 elderly patients with OIC. They found that the group with OIC had significantly higher total healthcare costs than the group without OIC ($p < .05$). Fully 16% of the total healthcare costs were attributable to OIC.

An estimated 100 million patients in the United States suffer with chronic pain including arthritis. The estimated cost in 2010 was $261 to $300 billion for healthcare, and lost productivity and wages was approximately another $250 billion. Just as many of the current costs of the opioid epidemic have not been accounted for, and even recognized, the future is likely to hold even more categories of conditions, social and political effects, and changes in physician's practices.

Bibliography

Centers for Disease Control and Prevention. (2015). *Worker Productivity Measures | Model | Workplace Health Promotion | CDC*. Workplace Health Promotion. Washington, DC: Centers for Disease Control and Prevention.

Council of Economic Advisers. (2017). *The underestimated cost of the opioid crisis*. Washington, DC: Council of Economic Advisers.

Florence, C. S., Zhou, C., Luo, F., & Xu, L. (2016). The economic burden of prescription opioid overdose, abuse and dependence in the United States, 2013. *Medical Care, 54*(10), 901–906. doi:10.1097/MLR.0000000000000625

Generations United. (2018). *Raising the children of the opioid epidemic—Solutions and support for grandfamilies*. Washington, DC: Generations United.

Gopelrud, E., Hodge, S., & Benham, T. (2019). A substance use cost calculator for U.S. employers with an emphasis on prescription pain medication misuse. *Journal of Occupational and Environmental Medicine, 59*(11), 1063–1071. doi:10.1097/JOM.0000000000001157

Huskamp, H. A., & Iglehart, J. K. (2016). Mental health and substance-use reforms—Milestones reached, challenges ahead. *The New England Journal of Medicine, 375*(7), 688–695. doi:10.1056/NEJMhpr1601861

Kampman, K., & Jarvis, M. (2015). American Society of Addiction Medicine (ASAM) national practice guideline for the use of medications in the treatment of addiction involving opioid use. *Journal of Addiction Medicine, 9*(5), 358–367. doi:10.1097/ADM.0000000000000166

Kane-Gill, S. L., Rubin, E. C., Smithburger, P. L., Buckley, M. S., & Dasta, J. F. (2014). The cost of opioid-related adverse drug events. *Journal of Pain and Palliative Care Pharmacotherapy, 28*(3), 282–293. doi:10.3109/15360288.2014.938889

Melanson, S. E. F., & Petrides, A. K. (2018). Economics of pain management testing. *The Journal of Applied Laboratory Medicine, 2*(4), 587–597.

National Institute on Drug Abuse. (2019). *Dramatic increases in maternal opioid use and neonatal abstinence syndrome*. North Bethesda, MD: National Institute on Drug Abuse.

Potter, J. S., Dreifuss, J. A., Marino, E. N., Provost, S. E., Dodd, D. R., Rice, L. S., ... Weiss, R. D. (2015). The multi-site prescription opioid addiction treatment study: 18-month outcomes. *Journal of Substance Abuse Treatment, 48*(1), 62–69. doi:10.1016/j.jsat.2014.07.009

Rettner, R. (2018). U.S. life expectancy dropped in 2017. Drug overdose deaths are a big reason why. Retrieved from https://www.livescience.com/64188-life-expectancy-decline-drug-overdose-deaths.html

Schulte, F., & Lucas, E. (2017, November 6). Liquid gold: Pain doctors soak up profits by screening urine for drugs. *Kaiser Health News*. Retrieved from https://khn.org/news/liquid-gold-pain-doctors-soak-up-profits-by-screening-urine-for-drugs/

U.S. Department of Health and Human Services—Assistant Secretary for Planning and Evaluation. (2019). *Use of medication-assisted treatment for opioid use disorders in employer-sponsored health insurance: Out-of-pocket costs*. Washington, DC: U.S. Department of Health and Human Services—Assistant Secretary for Planning and Evaluation.

Wan, Y., Corman, S., Gao, X., Liu, S., Patel, H., & Mody, R. (2015). Economic burden of opioid-induced constipation among long-term opioid users with noncancer pain. *American Health and Drug Benefits, 8*(2), 93–102.

3

Opioid Use Disorder

Opioid use disorder (OUD) has reached epidemic proportions in the United States. Approximately 25% of patients who have been prescribed opioids for chronic pain misuse them. In addition, 8% to 12% develop OUD. This chapter gives you an overview of OUD and how to recognize signs that a patient is suffering from OUD.

In this chapter, you will learn how to:

- List the *Diagnostic and Statistical Manual of Mental Disorders*, Fifth Edition (*DSM-5*; American Psychiatric Association [APA], 2013) requirements for making the diagnosis of OUD.
- List typical symptoms and behaviors associated with OUD.
- Understand the central nervous system (CNS) and physiologic mechanisms of addictive behavior.
- Compare OUD with other behavioral effects associated with opioid use.

OUD DEFINED

OUD is one of the clearly defined substance use disorders (SUD) in the *DSM-5*, the current edition of the APA's standard for diagnosing mental illness, including substance abuse and addiction. Prescription opioids are the most frequently misused class of prescription drugs in the United States.

The *DSM-5* recognizes substance-related disorders resulting from the use of many separate classes of drugs:

- Alcohol
- Caffeine
- Cannabis
- Inhalants
- Opioids
- Sedatives, hypnotics, anxiolytics
- Phencyclidine and other hallucinogens
- Stimulants
- Tobacco
- Other or unknown substances

While the pharmacological mechanisms of action for each class of drug are different, the activation of the brain's reward and motivation systems are similar across all the classes of substances.

OUD is a problematic pattern of use and behaviors that contributes to significant impairment or distress. Patients with OUD must feature a strong urge or craving for opioids, and physical, emotional, and psychological symptoms associated with withdrawal or sudden discontinuation of the opioids. Opioid use and cravings occur despite significant adverse effects, whether they be personal, psychosocial, family, and/or work related.

Complications of OUD include opioid overdose, often fatal if not treated in time with opioid antagonist rescue medication; progression to more potent or illicit forms of opioids; hepatitis C; HIV; family and marital disruption; and unemployment.

Signs and Symptoms of Opioid Intoxication

- Decreased perception of pain
- Euphoria
- Confusion
- Desire to sleep
- Nausea
- Constipation
- Miosis
- Bradycardia
- Hypotension
- Hypokinesis
- Head nodding
- Slurred speech
- Hypothermia

OUD DEFINED IN *DSM-5*

In 2006, a working group with the American Psychiatric Association revised the definitions and categorization of substance use disorders. The most recent version of the *DSM-5* was published in 2013.

OUD is defined as two or more of the following within a 12-month period:

- Using larger amounts of opioids or over a longer period than was intended
- Persistent desire to cut down or unsuccessful efforts to control use
- Great deal of time spent obtaining, using, or recovering from use
- Craving, or a strong desire or urge to use the substance
- Failure to fulfill major role obligations at work, school, or home due to recurrent opioid use
- Continued use despite recurrent or persistent social or interpersonal problems caused or exacerbated by opioid use
- Giving up or reducing social, occupational, or recreational activities due to opioid use
- Recurrent opioid use in physically hazardous situations
- Continued opioid use despite physical or psychological problems caused or exacerbated by its use
- Tolerance (marked increase in amount; marked decrease in effect)
- Withdrawal syndrome as manifested by cessation of opioids or use of opioids (or a closely related substance) to relieve or avoid withdrawal symptoms

Fast Facts

Tolerance and withdrawal criteria are not considered to be met for those taking opioids solely under appropriate medical supervision.

Severity of OUD is categorized as mild (presence of two or three symptoms), moderate (four or five symptoms), or severe (six or more symptoms).

Remission of OUD

- Early remission
    - None of the criteria for OUD have been met for at least 3 months but for less than 12 months (with the exception of craving, or a strong desire or urge to use opioids), but previously the full criteria for OUD were met to substantiate the diagnosis of OUD.

- Sustained remission
  - None of the criteria for OUD have been met at any time during a period of 12 months or longer (with the exception of craving, or a strong desire or urge to use opioids), but full criteria for OUD were previously met.

In 2018, the National Institute on Drug Abuse (NIDA) developed a simple list of 11 questions to ask patients to screen for OUD in emergency or primary care settings. The questions are based on the *DSM-5* criteria for OUD discussed earlier. Exhibit 3.1 is a simplified version of the NIDA-Modified ASSIST form (see Appendix B).

Exhibit 3.1

National Institute of Drug Abuse (NIDA) Simplified Screening for Opioid Use Disorder

Questions about your use of [name of opioid(s)] in the past 12 months (keep track of yes responses):

1. Have you often found that when you started using [name opioid(s)], you ended up taking more than you intended to?
2. Have you wanted to stop or cut down using or control your use of XX?
3. Have you spent a lot of time getting XX or using XX?
4. Have you had a strong desire or urge to use XX?
5. Have you missed work or school or often arrived late because you were intoxicated, high, or recovering from the night before?
6. Has your use of XX caused problems with other people such as with family members, friends, or people at work?
7. Have you had to give up or spend less time working, enjoying hobbies, or being with others because of your drug use?
8. Have you ever gotten high before doing something that requires coordination or concentration such as driving, boating, climbing a ladder, or operating heavy machinery?
9. Have you continued to use even though you knew that the drug caused you problems such as making you depressed, anxious, agitated, or irritable?
10. Have you found you needed to use much more drug to get the same effect that you did when you first started taking it?

(continued)

Exhibit 3.1

National Institute on Drug Abuse (NIDA) Simplified Screening for Opioid Use Disorder (*continued*)

11. When you reduced or stopped using, did you have withdrawal symptoms or felt sick when you cut down or stopped using (aches, shaking, fever, weakness, diarrhea, nausea, sweating, heart pounding, difficulty sleeping, or feeling agitated, anxious, irritable, or depressed)?

Count the number of yes answers to the questions above:

- Four or five: Moderate opioid use disorder
- Six or more: Severe opioid use disorder

Source: National Institutes of Drug Abuse. (2018). *Questions for identification of opioid use disorder based on DSM-5*. Retrieved from https://www.drugabuse.gov/nidamed-medical-health-professionals/discipline-specific-resources/initiating-buprenorphine-treatment-in-emergency-department/questions-identification-opioid-use-disorder-based-dsm-5.

REWARD AND MOTIVATION

All members of the opioid drug class share common pharmacological features as agonists of the *mu* opioid receptor. Opioids are highly addictive, with rapid progression to physiological dependence with tolerance and withdrawal.

Fast Facts

Opioids trigger the release of endorphins, your brain's feel-good neurotransmitters.

The activation of the CNS reward system is fundamental to the behaviors associated with OUD. Positive reinforcement is largely mediated by the indirect downstream activation of dopamine receptors, one of the main final common pathways of reward. High in the hierarchy of rewarding substances, opioids produce higher levels of positive reinforcement in both animal and human self-administration models than other drugs, except stimulants.

One of the important aspects of opioids, more than other addictive drugs, is negative reinforcement produced by opioid withdrawal.

Although the onset of withdrawal following opioid discontinuation varies with the half-life of the particular opioid, it produces a characteristic physiological syndrome with even brief abstinence or even a delay in dosing. Steady exposure to opioids can produce this process of neuroadaptation, leading to physiological dependence and withdrawal within as little as 4 to 8 weeks in opioid-naive individuals, and much faster with reinstatement after relapse in those with prior dependence. Opioid withdrawal includes activation of the locus coeruleus region of the brain with increased systemic sympathetic tone, which physiologically results in the classic withdrawal symptoms.

Withdrawal Symptoms

- Agitation
- Anxiety
- Muscle pains
- Increased tearing
- Trouble sleeping
- Runny nose
- Sweating
- Yawning
- Goose bumps
- Dilated pupils
- Diarrhea
- Fast heart rate
- High blood pressure
- Abdominal cramps
- Shakiness
- Cravings
- Sneezing

The progression of use often follows a pattern that maximizes drug bioavailability and effect.

The typical progression:
Oral prescription opioids → Inhaled prescription opioids → Inhaled heroin → Injection heroin

Inhalation can encompass either smoking or inhaling opioid smoke and nasal snorting of pulverized opioid tablets. Neither of these methods is as potent or efficient as injection, which maximizes bioavailability. This progression follows heroin's lower cost and higher potency.

Fast Facts

As tolerance to prescription opiates increases, and cost becomes prohibitive, the user will turn to lower cost and higher potency heroin.

CO-OCCURRING PSYCHIATRIC CONDITIONS

Patients with coexisting psychiatric conditions such as depression, anxiety, and PTSD may self-medicate with opioids, other drugs, and alcohol. Some individuals with prescription opioid dependence consume opioids to cope with emotional distress. Limited research examines the severity of the emotional distress and frequency of comorbid mood and anxiety disorders in this population.

In 2006, a study of psychiatric comorbidity and pain characteristics in patients entering a drug rehabilitation center identified comorbid OUD with an additional Axis I disorder in 14.7% of patients and comorbid polysubstance abuse/dependence with an additional Axis I disorder in 45.0% of patients. However, the study did not investigate the influence of comorbidity on the severity of either disorder and relied on patients entering drug rehabilitation, limiting the understanding of this population.

Examples of Axis I Disorders

- Anxiety disorders
- Panic disorders
- Social anxiety disorder
- PTSD
- Mood disorders
- Eating disorders
- Psychotic disorders
- Dissociative disorders

A recent population-based study found a statistically significant association between the past-year PTSD and polydrug misuse that included opioids.

Fast Facts

PTSD is highly prevalent in individuals with OUD using multiple substances.

In 2013, A cross-sectional study of prescription opioid dependence and comorbid mood and anxiety disorders reviewed 85 patients diagnosed with OUD after taking prescription opioids. The study found that 47.1% were also diagnosed with a mood or anxiety disorder.

Epidemiology of OUD

- About 3.8 million people in the United States aged 12 and older reported past-month misuse of a prescription pain medication in 2015.
- About half of these have the diagnosis of OUD.
- In the United States, over the past 20 years the vast majority of persons with OUD start by using prescription opioids.
- A significant proportion of these opioids have been appropriately prescribed by a provider, and illegally obtained through diversion.

Fast Facts

A study of young urban injection drug users revealed that 86% used illicit prescription opioids prior to using heroin. The opioids usually came from family, friends, or personal prescriptions.

RISK FACTORS FOR OUD

Risk factors for misuse of these medications and development of OUD are:

- Prior history of substance use disorder
- Certain demographic features (such as younger age)
- Severity of pain
- Higher daily opioid doses
- Concomitant prescription of certain psychiatric medications
- Prolonged duration of opioid prescription
- Co-occurring mental disorders

Typical risk factors such as stress, adversity, and exposure to substance use in family and peers tend to increase the risk for all substances rather than to opioid use or preference specifically. However, unique environmental influences differentially increase the risk of OUDs specifically.

Environmental influences that increase OUD risk include:

- Exposure to opioids as a specific class of substance, most importantly nonmedical use
- Exposure to medical opioid analgesics
- Use of opioids by family, peers, and other influential role models
- Permissive attitudes toward opioid use by influential role models
- Access to opioids as a specific substance class.

Fast Facts

The issue of ease of access, both for prescription opioids and for heroin, has been important in the genesis of the current epidemic.

At present, screening for opioid abuse includes:

- Assessment of premorbid and comorbid substance abuse
- Assessment of aberrant drug-related behaviors
- Risk factor stratification
- Utilization of opioid assessment screening tools

PHARMACOGENETICS AND OUD

Recent genetic studies have revealed that several specific loci are associated with opioid use and OUD. Specific allelic variants in various genes have been identified that seem to confer risk, including those genes coding for:

- Dopamine receptors and the dopamine transporter
- Opioid receptors
- Opioid neuropeptides
- Serotonin receptors and the serotonin transporter
- Cannabinoid receptors

For example, polymorphisms in the gene for the *mu*-opioid receptor (OPRM1) have been variably linked to differences in binding affinity and signaling efficiency, increased basal cortisol levels and opioid-mediated dynamic cortisol response, and differential analgesic effects of morphine; and some studies have found associations between these allelic variations and rates of opioid dependence, though others have not.

> **Fast Facts**
>
> *According to the American College of Obstetrics and Gynecology, 1% of pregnant women report nonmedical use of opioid pain medications. Pregnant women with OUD are at increased risk for adverse pregnancy outcomes including preterm labor, fetal death, growth restriction, and neonatal abstinence syndrome.*

TREATING OUD

The standard of care for treating OUD is medication-assisted treatment (MAT) that combines daily medically supervised administration of FDA-approved medications with behavioral therapy and counseling.

MAT is effective in:

- Facilitating recovery from OUD
- Preventing relapses
- Improving social and occupational functioning
- Reducing criminal behavior
- Reducing the spread of infectious diseases

The most effective treatment for withdrawal remains opioid replacement therapy with long-acting opioids such as methadone and buprenorphine. These medications prevent withdrawal symptoms and opioid cravings by continuous occupation of endogenous opioid receptors.

Brief Overview of Methadone

- Full agonist at the endogenous *mu* opioid receptor
- Mainstay of treatment for opioid addiction
- Long half-life and is ideally suited for once-daily oral dosing
- Carries the risks of respiratory depression
- The most commonly implicated prescription opioids in overdose deaths
- Shown to reduce mortality in patients with OUD by half
- Available only from federally regulated specialty clinics approved to prescribe and dispense the drug to patients who meet strict inclusion criteria

Brief Overview of Buprenorphine

- Partial agonist at the endogenous *mu* opioid receptor
- This partial activity prevents withdrawal but also blocks the action of full opioid agonists taken concomitantly
- Limited in its potential to cause sedation and respiratory depression, a safety advantage over methadone
- Traditionally available as a rapidly dissolving sublingual tablet or buccal film to deter IV injection of the drug
- Some formulations contain small amounts of the opioid antagonist naloxone (Narcan)
- Available by prescription from office-based physicians who are specially trained in treating OUD and have Drug Enforcement Administration (DEA) approval to prescribe it.

Recent studies, including a Cochrane meta-analysis, suggest that the retention with buprenorphine is lower than for methadone, but that buprenorphine may be associated with less drug use. Higher doses of buprenorphine are associated with better retention rates.

Fast Facts

Although both are effective, the choice between methadone and buprenorphine depends on individual patient factors such as proximity to treatment programs.

Whenever long-term opioid therapy is chosen, patients are encouraged to participate in educational programs as well as cognitive and behavioral therapy such as individual or group counseling and participation in self-help groups such as Narcotics Anonymous. Although maintenance therapy with methadone or buprenorphine can be tapered down over time, and in some cases discontinued altogether, most individuals require lifelong treatment as relapse rates are high.

OVERDOSE REVERSAL

Opioid overdose is a life-threatening emergency. Respiratory depression should be treated with naloxone, with respiratory support if necessary. Always utilize overdose as an opportunity to initiate addiction treatment. Make certain that patients on high doses of opioids or patients being treated for OUD, as well as household members of patients, have self-dosing naloxone immediately available for possible overdose.

Signs and Symptoms of Opioid Overdose

- Pin-point pupils
- Decreased heart rate
- Decreased body temperature
- Decreased breathing
- Altered level of consciousness
- Pulmonary edema
- Shock
- Death

MEDICALLY SUPERVISED WITHDRAWAL

Medically supervised opioid withdrawal, also known as detoxification, involves the administration of medication to reduce the severity of withdrawal symptoms. It is often a necessity but never sufficient treatment for OUDs. Medications used in the treatment of withdrawal may include buprenorphine, clonidine, and others for relief of symptoms. Medically supervised withdrawal is associated with high relapse rates ranging from 59% to more than 90% and poorer outcomes.

> **Fast Facts**
>
> *Emerging consensus supports the incorporation of relapse prevention medications such as buprenorphine and extended release naltrexone into comprehensive psychosocial treatment including counseling and family involvement.*

Bibliography

Ahmed, M., Haq, I. U., Faisal, M., Waseem, D., & Taqi, M. M. (2018). Implication of OPRM1 A118G polymorphism in opioids addicts in Pakistan: In vitro and in silico analysis. *Journal of Molecular Neuroscience, 65*(4), 472–479. doi:10.1007/s12031-018-1123-1

American College of Obstetricians and Gynecologists. (2017). *Opioid use and opioid use disorder in pregnancy.* ACOG Committee Opinion Number 711. Washington, DC: American College of Obstetricians and Gynecologists.

American Psychiatric Association. (2013). *Diagnostic and statistical manual of mental disorders, fifth edition.* Washington, DC: American Psychiatric Association.

Burns, L., & Teesson, M. (2002). Alcohol use disorders comorbid with anxiety, depression and drug use disorders. Findings from the Australian

National Survey of Mental Health and Well-Being. *Drug and Alcohol Dependence, 68*(3), 299–307. doi:10.1016/s0376-8716(02)00220-x

Diaper, A. M., Law, F. D., & Melichar, J. K. (2014). Pharmacological strategies for detoxification. *British Journal of Clinical Pharmacology, 77*(2), 302–314. doi:10.1111/bcp.12245

Gros, D. F., Milanak, M. E., Brady, K. T., & Back, S. E. (2013). Frequency and severity of comorbid mood and anxiety disorders in prescription opioid dependence. *The American Journal on Addictions, 22*(3), 261–265. doi:10.1111/j.1521-0391.2012.12008.x

Hasin, D. S., O'Brien, C. P., Auriacombe, M., Borges, G., Bucholz, K., Budney, A., ... Grant, B. F. (2013). *DSM-5* criteria for substance use disorders: Recommendations and rationale. *The American Journal of Psychiatry, 170*(8), 834–851. doi:10.1176/appi.ajp.2013.12060782

Hassan, A. N., & Le Foll, B. (2019). Polydrug use disorders in individuals with opioid use disorder. *Drug and Alcohol Dependence, 198*, 28–33. doi:10.1016/j.drugalcdep.2019.01.031

Katzman, J. G., Greenberg, N. H., Takeda, M. Y., & Moya Balasch, M. (2019). Characteristics of patients with opioid use disorder associated with performing overdose reversals in the community: An opioid treatment program analysis. *Journal of Addiction Medicine, 13*(2), 131–138. doi:10.1097/ADM.0000000000000461

Kaye, A. D., Jones, M. R., Kaye, A. M., Ripoll, J. G., Galan, V., Beakley, B. D., ... Manchikanti, L. (2017). Prescription opioid abuse in chronic pain: An updated review of opioid abuse predictors and strategies to curb opioid abuse: Part 1. *Pain Physician, 20*(2s), S93–S109.

Kreek, M. J., Levran, O., Reed, B., Schlussman, S. D., Zhou, Y., & Butelman, E. R. (2012). Opiate addiction and cocaine addiction: Underlying molecular neurobiology and genetics. *Journal of Clinical Investigation, 122*(10), 3387–3393. doi:10.1172/JCI60390

Lankenau, S. E., Teti, M., Silva, K., Jackson Bloom, J., Harocopos, A., & Treese, M. (2012). Initiation into prescription opioid misuse amongst young injection drug users. *International Journal of Drug Policy, 23*(1), 37–44. doi:10.1016/j.drugpo.2011.05.014

National Institute on Drug Abuse. (2018a). Prescription opioid use is a risk factor for heroin use. *NIDA News*. Retrieved from https://www.drugabuse.gov/publications/research-reports/relationship-between-prescription-drug-heroin-abuse/heroin-use-rare-in-prescription-drug-users

National Institute on Drug Abuse. (2018b). *Questions for identification of opioid use disorder based on DSM-5*. North Bethesda, MD: National Institute on Drug Abuse.

Nelson, E. C., Agrawal, A., Heath, A. C., Bogdan, R., Sherva, R., Zhang, B., ... Montgomery, G. W. (2016). Evidence of CNIH3 involvement in opioid dependence. *Molecular Psychiatry, 21*(5), 608–614. doi:10.1038/mp.2015.102

Passik, S. D., Hays, L., Eisner, N., & Kirsh, K. L. (2006). Psychiatric and pain characteristics of prescription drug abusers entering drug rehabilitation. *Journal of Pain and Palliative Care Pharmacotherapy, 20*(2), 5–13.

Schuckit, M. A. (2016). Treatment of opioid-use disorders. *The New England Journal of Medicine, 375*(4), 357–368. doi:10.1056/NEJMra1604339

Sharma, B., Bruner, A., Barnett, G., & Fishman, M. (2016). Opioid use disorders. *Child and Adolescent Psychiatric Clinics of North America, 25*(3), 473–487. doi:10.1016/j.chc.2016.03.002

Soyka, M. (2015). New developments in the management of opioid dependence: Focus on sublingual buprenorphine-naloxone. *Substance Abuse and Rehabilitation, 6*, 1–14. doi:10.2147/SAR.S45585

II

Overview of Cannabis

4
History and Legality of Cannabis

This chapter provides a brief history of medical cannabis use and the legal framework for the topics discussed throughout the following chapters. It charts the development and spread of cannabis in its various uses as fiber, food, and medicine as far back as 5,000 years ago. It also provides you, the healthcare provider, with the reassurances you need to discuss cannabis with your patients, and with the court rulings that protect your right to have these discussions even in states that do not currently allow legal medical cannabis.

In this chapter, you will learn how to:

- Compare and relate the historical medicinal uses of cannabis to modern resurgence in patient use of medical marijuana.
- Explain why there is a lack of clinical studies in medical marijuana use due to Schedule I classification of marijuana.
- Interpret the legal context in which cannabis can be discussed with a patient.
- Explain how states can have enacted medical marijuana laws even though it is recognized as a federally illegal substance.

TYPES OF CANNABIS

Cannabis, also commonly referred to as marijuana or hemp, is a genus of flowering plants in the family *Cannabaceae* that includes at least three species, *Cannabis sativa* L., *C. indica*, and *C. ruderalis*, differentiated by plant phenotypes and secondary metabolite profiles (terpene profiles). In practice, cannabis nomenclature is often used interchangeably among the three species. However, legally, hemp and marijuana are distinguished by their respective concentrations of the cannabidiol (CBD) delta-9-tetrahydrocannabinol (THC) found in the flowering tops and leaves. According to federal law, cannabis with 0.3% or less concentration of THC is not marijuana; it is industrial hemp.

C. sativa L. (Figure 4.1)

- Plants are gangly, at times stretching 20 feet tall
- Narrow, finger-shaped leaves and rangy buds
- Psychoactivity is more energetic high
- Stimulates talkativeness and nervousness
- Increases focus and creativity
- Increases serotonin
- Generally for day time use

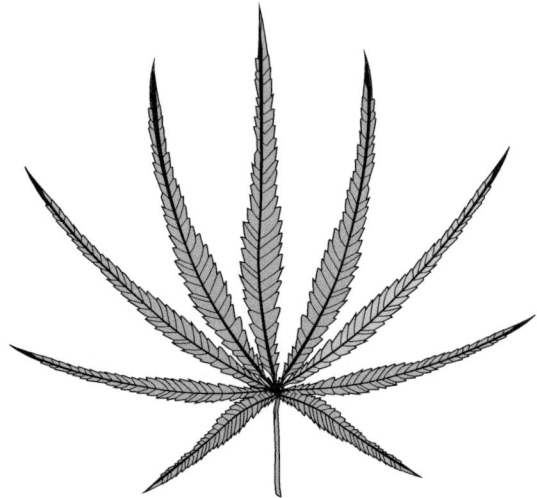

Figure 4.1 *C. sativa* leaf

C. indica (Figure 4.2)

- Plants are shorter and bushier
- Round leaves
- Psychoactivity is physical high commonly referred to as "couchlock"
- Increases mental and muscle relaxation
- Increases sleepiness
- Increases dopamine
- Generally for nighttime use

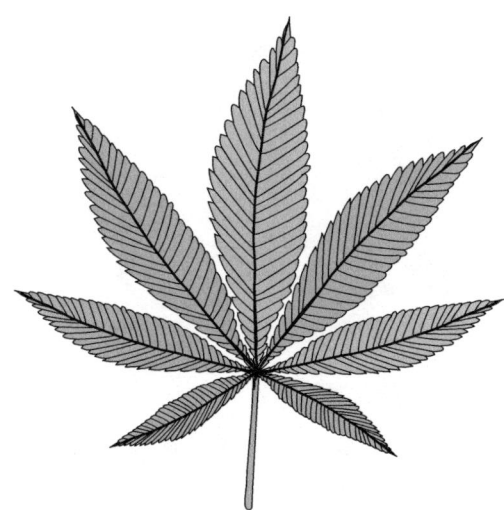

Figure 4.2 *C. indica* leaf

C. ruderalis (Figure 4.3)

- Plants are short and stalky
- Wide leaflets with a light green hue
- Contains low levels of THC
- Often contains high levels of CBD
- Traditionally used to create fast flowering strains when cross-bred with *C. sativa* strains

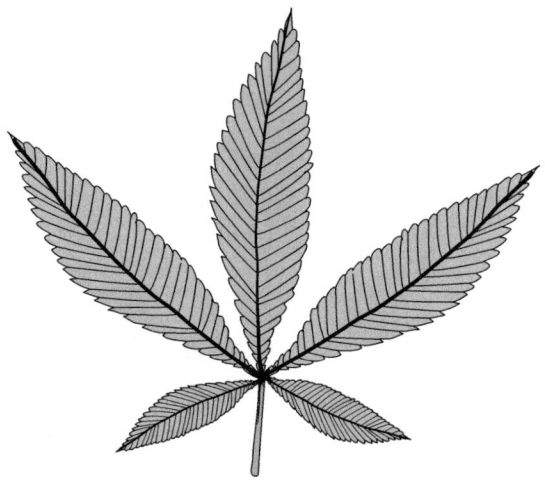

Figure 4.3 *C. ruderalis* leaf

The terms *sativa* and *indica* are, by and large, meaningless, as the plant in North America has been hybridized over the last 50 to 60 years. Though the terms are unreliable at predicting effects, they are now ingrained in the common lexicon, and we use them here with that forewarning.

Fast Facts

As a result of cannabis prohibition, recreational users selected THC-dominant strains that have more psychoactive properties than CBD. The result was the largest inadvertent breeding experiment, and CBD was largely eliminated from the majority of U.S. crops.

EARLY HISTORY OF CANNABIS USE

The ancient Chinese considered cannabis, called "ma," one of the 50 fundamental herbs and were the first to document its medicinal benefits over 4,700 years ago. The father of Chinese medicine, Shen-Nung, used ma to treat illnesses including gout, rheumatism, malaria, and constipation. In India, Ayurvedic medicinal traditions used the drug extensively. The Egyptians used it in suppositories and to relieve eye pain. The Greeks made wine steeped with cannabis, which they used to treat inflammation and ear problems (see Figure 4.4 for a timeline of cannabis use).

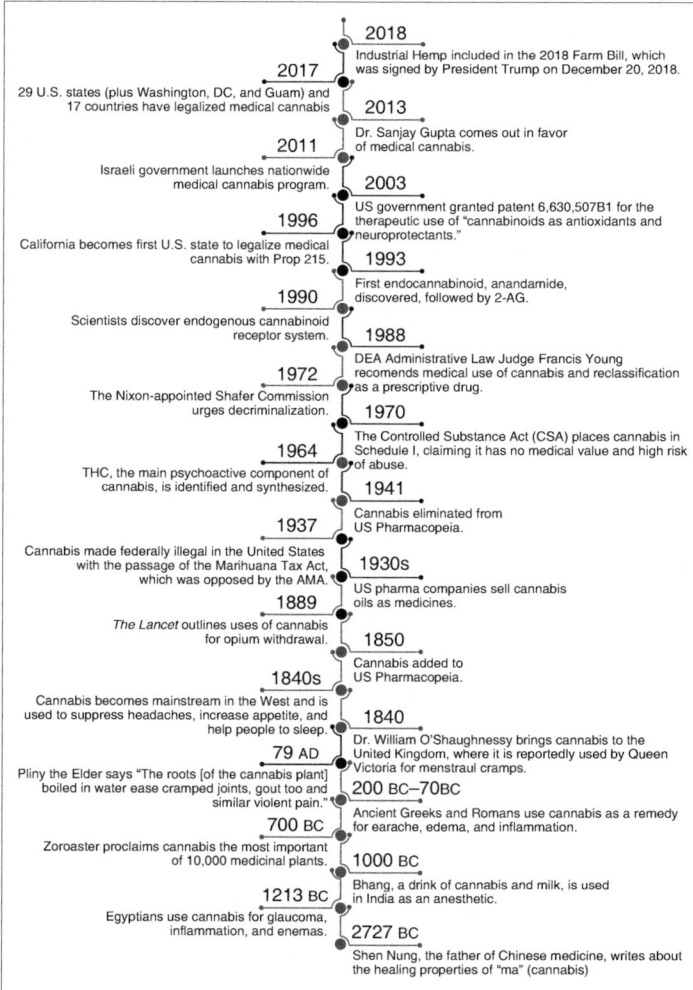

Figure 4.4 Cannabis timeline.

2-AG, 2-arachidonoylglycerol; AMA, American Medical Association; DEA, Drug Enforcement Administration; THC, tetrahydrocannabinol.

Ailments Treated Using Cannabis

- Suppositories for hemorrhoids
- Relieve eye pain
- Chronic pain
- Insomnia
- Inflammation in the ears
- Headaches and migraines
- Gastrointestinal disorders
- Increase appetite
- Reduce nausea
- Muscle spasms
- Anticonvulsant
- Analgesic
- Anti-inflammatory

U.S. PROHIBITION

In 1900, *C. indica* was most often prescribed for pain and insomnia. In 1898, aspirin was synthesized from willow bark, and shortly thereafter the first barbiturates were also produced as pills. In the 1930s, Harry Anslinger proposed the Marihuana Tax Act to Congress. The Act did not criminalize the possession or medicinal use of hemp, marijuana, or cannabis, but included penalty and enforcement provisions to which marijuana, cannabis, or hemp handlers were subject. Violation of these procedures could result in a fine of up to $2,000 and 5 years imprisonment. In addition, every person who sold, dealt in, dispensed, or gave away marijuana had to register with the Internal Revenue Service and pay a special occupational tax.

The use of marijuana, as both a recreational and medicinal drug, began to dissipate. According to U.S. Customs and Border Protection, the Marihuana Tax Act of 1937 intended to stop only the use of the plant as a recreational drug. In practice, though, industrial hemp was caught up in anti-marijuana legislation, making hemp importation and commercial production in this country less economical. Scientific research and medical testing of cannabis virtually disappeared. By 1941, the Marihuana Tax Act had imposed such a burden that doctors stopped prescribing cannabis. It was dropped from the American Pharmacopeia in 1941. In 1970, marijuana was classified and restricted on par with narcotics and new, tighter laws were enacted.

PRESENT LEGAL STATUS OF CANNABIS

Marijuana is currently classified as a Schedule I drug under the Controlled Substances Act (CSA; see Table 4.1).
Schedule I drugs are defined as

- Drugs or other substances that have a high potential for abuse.
- Drugs or other substances that have no currently accepted medical use in treatment in the United States.
- There is a lack of accepted safety for use of the drugs or other substances under medical supervision.

Since 1972, cannabis has been classified as a Schedule I drug under the U.S. CSA because the U.S. Drug Enforcement Agency considers it to have "no accepted medical use."

However, as of July 2019, 33 of the 50 U.S. states and the District of Columbia have recognized the medical benefits of cannabis and have decriminalized its medical use.

States With Medical Marijuana Laws

- Alaska
- Arizona
- Arkansas
- California
- Colorado
- Connecticut
- Delaware
- District of Columbia
- Florida
- Hawaii
- Illinois
- Louisiana
- Maine
- Maryland
- Massachusetts
- Michigan
- Minnesota
- Missouri
- Montana
- Nevada
- New Hampshire
- New Jersey
- New Mexico
- New York
- North Dakota
- Ohio
- Oklahoma
- Oregon
- Pennsylvania
- Rhode Island
- Utah
- Vermont
- Washington
- West Virginia

Table 4.1

Examples of Drug Classifications in the United States

Schedule	Description	Examples
Schedule I	Drugs with no currently accepted medical use and a high potential for abuse. They are the most dangerous drugs of all the drug schedules with potentially severe psychological or physical dependence.	Heroin Lysergic acid diethylamide (LSD) Marijuana (cannabis) Methylenedioxymethamphetamine Methaqualone Peyote
Schedule II	Drugs with a high potential for abuse, with use potentially leading to severe psychological or physical dependence. These drugs are also considered dangerous.	Cocaine Methamphetamine Methadone Meperidine Oxycodone Fentanyl Morphine Methylphenidate Hydromorphone Combination products with less than 15 mg of hydrocodone per dosage unit
Schedule III	Drugs with a moderate to low potential for physical and psychological dependence. Schedule III drugs abuse potential is less than Schedules I and II, but more than Schedule IV.	Ketamine Anabolic steroids Testosterone Combination products with less than 90 mg of codeine per dosage unit and buprenorphine
Schedule IV	Drugs with a low potential for abuse and low risk of dependence.	Alprazolam Carisoprodol Propoxyphene Tramadol Benzodiazepines Diazepam Zolpidem
Schedule V	Drugs with a lower potential for abuse than Schedule IV and consist of preparations containing limited quantities of certain narcotics. Schedule V drugs are generally used for antidiarrheal, antitussive, and analgesic purposes.	Cannabidiol Ezogabine Attapulgite Difenoxin and atropine Cough preparations with less than 200 mg of codeine per 100 mL

Source: Drug Enforcement Agency.

The approved list of conditions/diseases, and the other laws/rules regarding the possession and cultivation of medical marijuana differ by state. In addition, 11 of the 50 U.S. states and the District of Columbia have legalized recreational cannabis use for adults 21 years of age and above, with varying rules and regulations.

Approved Ailments Varies by State

- Alzheimer's disease
- Amyotrophic lateral sclerosis
- Anorexia
- Arthritis
- Autism
- Cachexia
- Cancer
- Chronic pain
- Crohn's disease
- Glaucoma
- Hepatitis C
- HIV/AIDS
- Intractable pain
- Migraine
- Nausea
- PTSD
- Seizures
- Spasticity
- Tourette's syndrome
- Traumatic brain Injury
- Terminal conditions

In 2009, Senators Ron Paul and Barney Frank introduced the Industrial Hemp Farming Act to amend the definition of "marihuana" [sic] in the CSA to clarify the difference between hemp and marijuana. Industrial hemp was included in the 2018 Farm Bill, which was signed by the president on December 20, 2018. This legislature removed industrial hemp from the Schedule I drug classification per section 10113 of the Farm Bill.

Fast Facts

Industrial hemp is defined as containing less than 0.3% THC. Legally grown hemp is the source of CBD products on the market today.

With the declassification of industrial hemp, products that contain CBD derived from legal hemp are now federally legal. This bill moved CBD to Schedule V drug classification. The bill also removes restrictions on the sale, transport, and possession of hemp-derived products, so long as those items are produced in a manner consistent with the law. This change in the way hemp is regulated opens research options regarding CBD, but there are still areas of uncertainty regarding how research-grade cannabis can be obtained. Currently, research-grade cannabis must be obtained from the University of Mississippi School of Pharmacy's National Center for Natural Products Research due to the Schedule I status of cannabis. Additional guidance will be required from the Food and Drug Administration (FDA), Drug Enforcement Administration (DEA), and National Institute on Drug Abuse (NIDA) on this policy and how the farm bill will change the research process involving hemp-derived CBD.

FEDERAL LEGAL FRAMEWORK

This outline list provides an introductory overview of relevant federal cannabis regulations. Many sections included here may not be relevant to medical application but are important for people to consider before deciding to use medical cannabis.

CSA (21 USCA 801, et seq.) (1970)

- Marijuana is a Schedule I drug.
- Federal preemption of state laws is in "direct conflict" with the CSA

Ogden, Cole, and Wilkinson Memos

Guidance for prosecutorial discretion—not federal legalization

- **Ogden Memo (2009)**—First guidance from the Department of Justice on medical marijuana enforcement
- **Cole Memos (2011–2014)**—Established the eight Department of Justice priorities on drug enforcement and focus at the federal level.

  - Distribution of marijuana to minors
  - Revenue from the sale of marijuana from going to criminal enterprises, gangs, and cartels
  - Diversion of marijuana from states where it is legal under state law in some form to other states

- State-authorized marijuana activity from being used as a cover or pretext for the trafficking of other illegal drugs or other illegal activity
- Violence and the use of firearms in the cultivation and distribution of marijuana
- Drugged driving and the exacerbation of other adverse public health consequences associated with marijuana use
- Growing of marijuana on public lands and the attendant public safety and environmental dangers posed by marijuana production on public lands
- Marijuana possession or use on federal property (Cole, 2014)

- **Wilkinson Memo (2014)**—Extended Department of Justice enforcement priorities to tribal lands.

The Rohrabacher–Farr Amendment (2014)

More recently known as the Rohrabacher–Blumenauer Amendment, it is legislation first introduced by U.S. Reps. Maurice Hinchey, Dana Rohrabacher, and Sam Farr in 2003. It prohibited the Justice Department from spending funds to interfere with the implementation of state medical cannabis laws. The amendment does not change the legal status of cannabis and must be renewed each fiscal year to remain in effect. There is one unpublished case in California where the federal court upheld the Rohrabacher–Farr Amendment and extended the protection to recreational cannabis.

In addition to these recent developments, the U.S. government has set a precedent for patenting cannabis and cannabis-related inventions. For example, U.S. Pat. No. 6,630,507 issued on October 7, 2003, and assigned to the United States of America, is directed to methods of treating diseases caused by oxidative stress by administering therapeutically effective amounts of a CBD cannabinoid from cannabis that has substantially no binding to the N-methyl-D-aspartate (NMDA) receptor, wherein the CBD acts as an antioxidant and neuroprotectant. The U.S. Patent and Trademark Office confirmed that officials now accept and process patent applications for individual varieties of cannabis, along with innovative medical uses for the plant and other associated inventions.

Fast Facts

In 2018, Gallup reported that 66% of people supported marijuana legalization in the United States.

Despite the conflicting official positions within the federal government, many states recognize that cannabis provides substantial benefits for medical and recreational uses. As of the November 2018 elections, cannabis has been legalized or decriminalized in 33 states to treat a variety of state-approved conditions. However, healthcare professionals in all states are not able to discuss cannabis with patients, due to Schedule I classification, until the ruling by the Ninth Circuit Court in the 2002 case of *Conant v. Walters*.

CONANT V. WALTERS—HEALTHCARE PROVIDER RECOMMENDATIONS

After California and Arizona decriminalized medical marijuana in 1996, the Federal Department of Justice and the Department of Health and Human Services sent a policy to federal, state, and local practitioner associations cautioning physicians who "intentionally provide their patients with oral or written statements in order to enable them to obtain controlled substances in violation of federal law risk revocation of their DEA prescription authority" (*Conant v. Walters*, 2002).

In 2002, the Ninth Circuit affirmed an order permanently instructing the federal government not to:

- Revoke a physician's license to prescribe controlled substances.
- Conduct an investigation of a physician that might lead to such revocation, where the basis for the government action would be solely the physician's "recommendation" of the use of medical marijuana, on First Amendment grounds.

As a result of the ruling by the Ninth Circuit, physicians are protected by the First Amendment in all states to discuss the pros and cons of medical marijuana with patients and issue written or oral recommendations to use marijuana within a bona fide doctor–patient relationship without fear of legal reprisal. And this is so, regardless of whether the physician anticipates that the patient will, in turn, use this recommendation to obtain marijuana in violation of federal law. On the other hand, the physician may not actually prescribe or dispense marijuana to a patient or recommend it in writing in a manner such that the patient will use the recommendation like a prescription to obtain marijuana. There have been no such criminal or administrative proceedings against doctors to date.

Fast Facts

States with medical marijuana laws require the recommendation from a physician, or nurse practitioner in some states, before a patient can obtain and use cannabis for medicinal purposes.

Doctors and Prescribers MAY:

- Discuss, fully and candidly, the risks and benefits of medical marijuana with patients.
- Recommend (or approve, endorse, suggest, or advise, etc.), in accordance with their medical judgment, marijuana for patient use.
- Record in their patients' charts discussions about and recommendations of medical marijuana.
- Sign government forms or inform state or local officials that they have recommended medical marijuana for patients.
- Testify in court or through written declaration about recommending medical marijuana for their patients.
- Educate themselves about the medical benefits of marijuana, its various clinical applications, and different routes of ingestion.

Doctors and Prescribers MAY NOT:

- Prescribe medical marijuana. This includes writing a recommendation on an Rx form.
- Assist patients in obtaining marijuana.
- Cultivate or possess marijuana for patient use.
- Physically assist patients in using marijuana.
- Recommend marijuana without a justifiable medical cause.

ADDITIONAL LEGAL CONSIDERATIONS FOR PATIENTS

No matter the current state regulations, marijuana is federally classified as a Schedule I drug, so cannabis users are not a protected class. Drug testing is permitted and employers can terminate employment for having THC in their blood or urine. This is regardless of a patient having a state-approved medical marijuana card or if using cannabis has no effect on their job performance. Rightful termination may depend on whether the employment contract contains a provision with the requirement of following all federal laws and refraining from partaking illegal drugs.

Additional Considerations

- Patients cannot cross state borders with medical marijuana
- Risk of driving under the influence
- Federal offense to possess or use marijuana in national parks or on military property
- Insurance plans do not cover medical marijuana patient costs

Reference

Cole, J. M. (2014). *Memorandum for all United States attorneys: Guidance regarding marijuana related financial crimes*. Washington, DC: U.S. Department of Justice, Office of the Deputy Attorney General.

Bibliography

Agriculture Improvement Act of 2018, H.R.2, 115th Con. (2018).
Brandon Coats V. Dish Network, LLC. 350 P.3d 849 (Colo. 2015).
Clarke, R. C., & Merlin, M. D. (2013). *Cannabis: Evolution and ethnobotany*. Berkeley: University of California Press.
Conant v. Walters, 309 F.3d 629 (9th Cir. 2002).
Constitution of the United States of America: Analysis and Interpretation. Article VI—Prior Debts, National Supremacy, and Oaths of Office. (2017). Washington, DC: U.S. Government Publishing Office.
H. Amdt. 748 to H.R. 1866. (2013–2014). Washington, DC: 113th Congress.
H.R. 1866. (2009). Washington, DC: 111th Congress, 1st Session.
John P. Walters, Et Al V. Dr. Marcus Conant, Et Al. F. 3d 309, 639 (9th Cir. 2003).
Murray, R. M., Morrison, P. D., Henquet, C., & Forti, M. (2007). Cannabis, the mind and society; The hash realities. *Nature Reviews Neuroscience, 8*, 885–895. doi:10.1038/nrn2253
National Conference of State Legislatures. (2019). *State medical marijuana laws*. Retrieved from http://www.ncsl.org/research/health/state-medical-marijuana-laws.aspx
National Institute on Drug Abuse. (2018). *Information on marijuana farm contract*. Bethesda, MD: National Institute on Drug Abuse.
Ogden, D. W. (2009). *Memorandum for selected United States attorneys: Investigation and prosecutions in states authorizing the medical use of marijuana*. Washington, DC: U.S. Department of Justice, Office of the Deputy Attorney General.
United States Department of Agriculture—Natural Resources Conservation Service. (2017). *Classification | USDA Plants*. Retrieved from plants.usda.gov

The United States of America as Represented by the Department of Health and Human Services. (1999). *Cannabinoids as antioxidants and neuroprotectants* (US6630507 B1).

United States of America v. Steve McIntosh. F. 3d 833, 1163, 1176 (9th Cir. 2016).

U.S.C. Title 21. Chapter 13, Subchapter I. Sec. 802—Definitions. (2016). Washington, DC: U.S. Government Publishing Office.

U.S.C. Title 21. Chapter 13, Subchapter I. Sec. 812—Schedules of controlled substances. (2016). Washington, DC: U.S. Government Publishing Office.

U.S.C. Title 7. Sec. 5490—Legitimacy of industrial hemp research. (2016). Washington, DC: U.S. Government Publishing Office.

U.S. Customs and Border Protection. (2015). *Did you know... Marijuana was once a legal cross-border import?* Washington, DC: U.S. Department of Homeland Security.

U.S. Legal. (2019). *Marijuana tax act law and legal definition.* Retrieved from https://definitions.uslegal.com/m/marijuana-tax-act%20/

Warf, B. (2014). High points: An historical geography of cannabis. *Geographical Review, 104*(4), 414–438. doi:10.1111/j.1931-0846.2014.12038.x

Wilkinson, M. (2014). *Memorandum: Policy statement regarding marijuana issues in Indian Country.* Washington, DC: U.S. Department of Justice, Executive Office for United States Attorneys.

5

Overview of the Endocannabinoid System

The endocannabinoid system (ECS) is involved in maintaining homeostasis, neuroprotection, and other regulatory functions. This chapter charts how the 1964 discovery of the cannabinoids delta-9-tetrahydrocannabinol (THC) and cannabidiol (CBD) led to the 1988 discovery of the ECS.

In this chapter, you will learn how to:

- Summarize the function of the ECS in the regulation of the body.
- Identify the physiological reason cannabinoids do not cause overdose deaths.
- Understand the similarities between endogenous and exogenous cannabinoids.

DISCOVERY OF THE ECS

The chemistry of cannabis remained a mystery until 1964. Raphael Mechoulam, PhD, then a 34-year-old biochemistry graduate student at the Weizmann Institute, and Yehiel Gaoni, PhD, employed a new separation technology to isolate the two most prevalent compounds of the plant: CBD and the psychoactive molecule delta-9-THC.

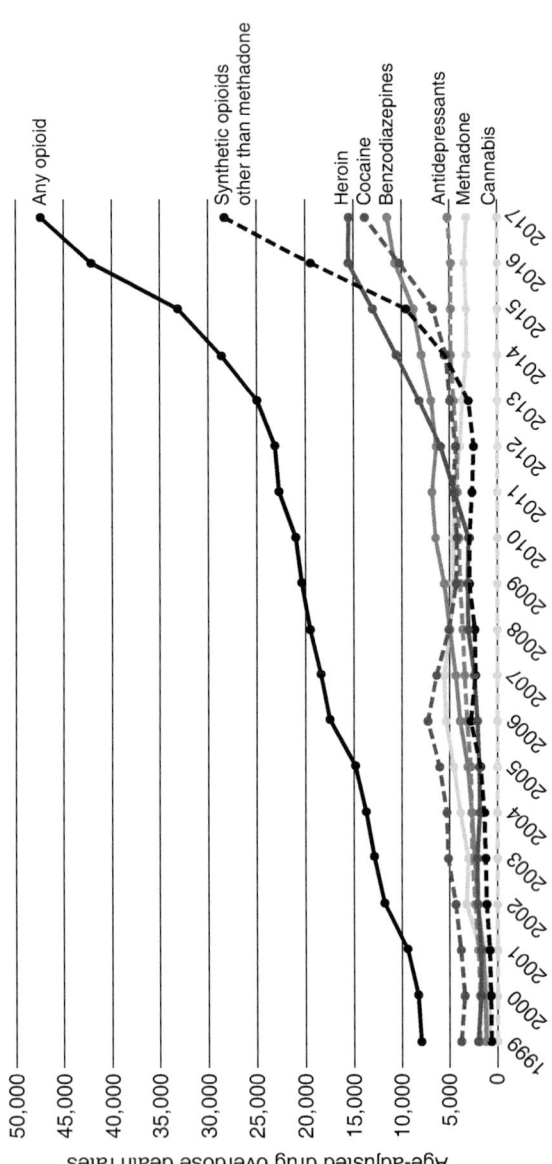

Figure 5.1 National drug overdose deaths, all ages, 1999–2017.
Source: Data from CDC WONDER.

In 1988, an American chemist, Allyn Howlett, PhD, located a large grouping of receptors in the brain that responded to THC. There are no receptors in the cardiac and respiratory centers of the brainstem, the areas that shut down the heart and lungs in cases of overdose. This is the physiological reason why, to date, there have been no reported deaths from a cannabis overdose.

Fast Facts

It is estimated that the average human would have to smoke 1,500 pounds of cannabis in 15 minutes to reach fatal levels.

Densest Receptor Concentrations in the Brain

- Cortex
- Cerebellum
- Hippocampus
- Basal ganglia

Brain Functions Affected by ECS

- Movement
- Emotions
- Memory
- Pain
- Pleasure
- Reproduction

In 1992, Mechoulam, in collaboration with NIMH research fellow William Devane and Dr. Lumir Hanus, found a novel neurotransmitter, a naturally occurring endocannabinoid that attaches to the same mammalian brain-cell receptors as THC. They decided to call it "anandamide," deriving from the Sanskrit word for bliss (Figure 5.2).

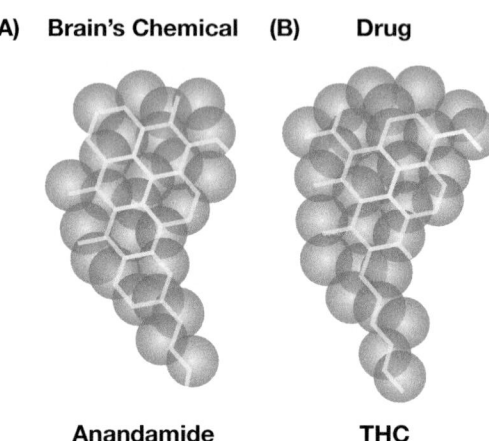

Figure 5.2 Comparison of (A) anandamide (AEA) and (B) THC molecular structures.

Just like THC, anandamide (AEA) is thought to intensify sensory experience, stimulate appetite, temporarily blot out short-term memory, and create feelings of pleasure. Shortly after, the lab identified another brain chemical that mimics CBD, 2-arachidonoylglycerol (2-AG). Both are synthesized on demand from acids in cell membranes (Figure 5.3).

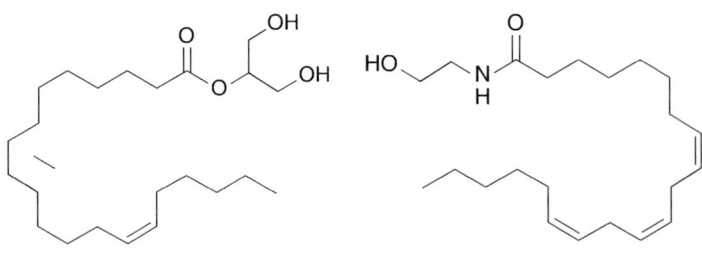

Figure 5.3 (A) Arachidonoylglycerol (2-AG) and (B) anandamide molecular structures.

THC, tetrahydrocannabinol.

Endocannabinoids Found in the Body

- AEA attaches to the same receptors as THC.
- 2-AG attaches to the same receptors as CBD.

This led to the discovery of a galaxy of endocannabinoid receptors that extends into every organ, gland, immune cell, and connective tissue. Receptors in the brain are known as cannabinoid receptors type 1 (CB1); those in the periphery are called cannabinoid receptors type 2 (CB2). Many tissues contain both CB1 and CB2 receptors, each responsible for a different action.

Fast Facts

Endocannabinoids, AEA, and 2-AG are endogenous lipids that are synthesized on demand from acids in cell membranes versus classical neurotransmitters that are synthesized in advance and stored in synaptic vesicles.

EVOLUTION OF THE ECS

By tracing the metabolic pathways of THC, scientists found a unique and hitherto unknown molecular signaling system that is involved in regulating a broad range of biological functions. They called it "the ECS," after the plant that led to its detection. The name suggests that the plant came first, but in fact, as Dr. John McPartland has explained, this ancient, internal signal system started evolving over 600 million years ago (long before cannabis appeared) when sponges were the most complex life form. The ECS receptor system is present in all animals.

The largest receptor system in the human body, the ECS functions are involved throughout all body systems and all hierarchical levels of biological organization. Endocannabinoids are also found at the intersection of the body's various systems, which allow different cell types to communicate. When an injury occurs, endocannabinoids decrease the release of activators and sensitizers from the injured tissue, stabilize nerve cells by opening potassium channels to prevent excessive firing, and calm immune cells in the area to slow the release of inflammatory substances.

ECS Regulates

- Aversive memory extinction
- Hypothalamic–pituitary–adrenal (HPA) axis modulation
- Immunomodulation
- Wake and sleep cycles
- Blood pressure
- Bone density
- Tumor surveillance
- Reproduction
- Neuroprotection

In the last 30 years, new pharmaceuticals have been developed to activate various receptor systems. Antihistamines, for example, initially targeted receptors in the nasal passages, but when additional histamine receptors were discovered in the digestive system a class of drugs called Histamine-2 (H2) were developed to target and treat gastric illnesses. Underproduction of dopamine is connected to Parkinson's disease; overproduction is related to schizophrenia. Serotonin, which mimics the psychedelic compounds in psilocybin mushrooms, mitigates depression.

WHY THE ECS IS NOT TAUGHT IN MEDICAL SCHOOLS

Cannabis' Schedule I status is the reason that no research institution has ever administered AEA to a human being. This is also one of the reasons why the ECS is not taught in medical schools; it makes little practical sense to spend time educating students about a bodily system that can only be treated by illegal compounds.

Fast Facts

The ECS is not taught in the traditional medical curriculum. A 2013 survey found that 87% of medical schools do not include the ECS as part of their medical curriculum.

Other countries are taking the lead by deploying cannabis to treat illnesses that have eluded modern medicine. In the last decade, Israel has built the world's largest state-supported medical cannabis program. Though it has not been widely advertised internationally, the program currently allows each of the 30,000-plus patients in it to receive 10 to 100 grams per month depending on the severity of the patient's condition. The monthly cost to a patient is fixed at roughly $100 and is reimbursed by Israeli National Health Insurance.

OVERVIEW OF THE ECS

The ECS functions are involved throughout all body systems and all hierarchical levels of biological organization. The ECS plays a key role in synaptic communication in the central nervous system (CNS). Cannabinoid receptors are the most common G-protein-coupled receptors in the CNS, with the highest densities in the cerebellum, hippocampus, cerebral cortex, and amygdaloid nucleus. Cannabinoid receptors also represent the second most common G-protein-coupled receptors in the body. The ECS regulates neuronal excitability and inflammation in pain circuits and cascades.

ECS Receptors Effect

- Mood and emotional responses
- Cognition
- Plasticity
- Motor functions
- Growth and development
- Learning and memory
- Eating and food drive
- Pain signaling and interpretation

Cannabinoids, both endogenous and exogenous, coordinate intracellular biochemistry, intercellular communication, and all body systems. Endocannabinoids have affected every biological oscillator or pacemaker cell investigated, including circadian rhythms, rhythmical variations in blood pressure known as Traube–Hering waves, peristalsis slow waves, EKG, and EEG rhythms.

The ECS consists of cannabinoid receptors, endogenous ligands known as endocannabinoids along with their transport mechanisms, and endocannabinoid metabolizing enzymes. The system functions as a self-regulating, harm-reduction system, influencing multiple physiologic processes in the human body in response to oxidative and physiologic stress (see also Table 5.1).

Fast Facts

Cannabis is known to be useful in eliminating painful memories in patients suffering from PTSD.

Table 5.1

Health Benefits of Endocannabinoid System Treatments

Seizure control	Studies show that cannabis reduces seizure frequency in adults and children and enhances anticonvulsant activity of traditional seizure medications.
Reduced anxiety	Cannabis acts on GABA receptors that activate the parasympathetic nervous system, reducing the fight-or-flight response and inducing a state of calm.
Bronchodilation	Although it seems counterintuitive, cannabinoids aid in bronchodilation and research teams are developing asthma treatments with cannabis.
Neuroprotection	Cannabinoids are successfully used as neuroprotectants in a range of conditions including MS, Alzheimer's disease, TBI, Parkinson's disease, ALS, and Huntington's disease.
Pain management	Over 300 studies have shown that cannabinoids can help patients with chronic pain, including 36 double-blind randomized controlled clinical trials.
Decreased inflammation	Cannabis has 20 times the anti-inflammatory potency of aspirin, and twice that of hydrocortisone—with minor adverse side effects when compared with mainstream medications.
Cancer care	Therapies with cannabis are effective in managing the adverse side effects of cancer treatment, while cannabinoids affect key cell signaling pathways that affect cancer cell survival and proliferation.
Reduced PTSD symptoms	Cannabis helps reprioritize painful memories/night terrors, reduce anxiety and fear response, and improve sleep for patients suffering from PTSD.
Migraine relief	Users of cannabis show a reduced frequency of migraines, and manipulation of CB2 receptors is a potential new target for developing migraine treatments.
Sleep aid	Anecdotal reports show that cannabis is effective in helping patients get to sleep faster, stay asleep longer, and feel well rested without the morning grogginess associated with sleeping pills.
Appetite stimulant	Cannabis functions as an appetite stimulant, helping patients suffering from chemotherapy side effects or a range of illnesses affecting appetite such as anorexia or ALS.
Tumor reduction	Cannabinoids prevent blood vessels from feeding tumors. Animal studies show that cannabinoids also slow angiogenesis and decrease metastasis in multiple tumor types.

(continued)

Table 5.1

Health Benefits of Endocannabinoid System Treatments (*continued*)

Ease GI disorders	Cannabinoids modulate actions of the gastrointestinal (GI) tract. Clinical and anecdotal data support cannabinoid therapy to help manage Crohn's disease, ulcerative colitis, IBS, and other GI illnesses.
Pain relief	Nearly 40 preclinical and clinical trials have shown that low-dose cannabis relieves neuropathic pain. Patients with arthritis and myofascial pain often seek pain relief with cannabis.

CB2, cannabinoid receptor type 2; ALS, amyotrophic lateral sclerosis; GABA, gamma aminobutyric acid; GI, gastrointestinal; IBS, irritable bowel syndrome; MS, multiple sclerosis; TBI, traumatic brain injury.

A network of endocannabinoid receptors weaves throughout the CNS and immune systems and within tissues including the brain, gastrointestinal system, reproductive system, spleen, endocrine system, and heart and circulatory system. Endocannabinoids serve as primary messengers across nerve synapses and signal neurons to communicate with each other. They modulate the flow of neurotransmitters, keeping the nervous system running smoothly. They affect circadian rhythms, rhythmical variations in blood pressure, peristalsis slow waves, and EKG and EEG rhythms.

ENDOCANNABINOIDS

Endocannabinoids are endogenous lipids that engage cannabinoid receptors. The first discovered and best-characterized endocannabinoids are arachidonoyl ethanolamide (anandamide) and 2-AG. Though they have a different molecular structure from THC and CBD, the molecules produced by the brain mirror the cannabinoids on the plant; both fit into the binding sites on cannabinoid receptors. Their precursors are present in lipid membranes. Upon demand (typically by activation of certain G-protein-coupled receptors or by depolarization), endocannabinoids are liberated in one or two rapid enzymatic steps and released into the extracellular space immediately, in contrast to other neurotransmitters that are synthesized ahead of time and stored in synaptic vesicles. The efficacy of the endogenous cannabinoids varies—2-AG is a high-efficacy agonist for both CB1 and CB2 receptors, however AEA is a low-efficacy agonist at CB1 receptors and a very low-efficacy agonist at CB2 receptors. Thus, in systems with low receptor expression or when receptors couple weakly to signaling pathways AEA can antagonize the effects of more efficacious agonists.

ECS RECEPTORS

Cannabinoid receptors are the densest receptors in the brain, denser than opiate or nicotinic receptors. The network constantly relays information about various states of cells, tissues, and organs. In the nervous system alone, cannabinoid receptors govern nerve transmission, memory, mood, emotion, pain perception, feeding, reproduction, metabolism, nerve protection (including nerve death caused by glutamate toxicity), as well as nervous system adaptability and brain development.

The two primary cannabinoid receptors, known as CB1 and CB2, differ in terms of where they are located and what they do.

CB1 Receptors

- Primarily located in the CNS
- Modulate neurotransmitter release
- Affect many brain functions including movement, anxiety, stress, fear, pain, appetite, reward, and motor control
- Causes psychoactivity when the CB1 receptor is activated

In the brain, much CB1 activity occurs in the nervous system at synapses. Because of their high densities, CB1 receptors are responsible for the effects of cannabis on short-term memory, cognition, mood and emotion, muscle motor function, pain perception, and nerve protection.

CB2 Receptors

- Located in the interstitium including blood plasma as well as immune system organs such as the spleen, tonsils, and lymphatics
- Controls the release of cytokines—immunoregulatory proteins—that are linked to inflammation during illness or after injury
- Involved with wound repair and fibrogenesis
- Upregulated in all tissues in response to injury or inflammation
- CB2 receptor activation causes no psychoactivity

CB1 and CB2 receptor densities in the nervous system vary significantly depending on the biologic state of the organism. In the connective tissue, fluctuations of cannabinoid receptor populations are as much as 25-fold. The ECS is a fluid, dynamic, and unstable system, and when functioning properly, receptor levels of endocannabinoids constantly adjust and adapt to internal and external microenvironments.

Locations of CB1 Receptors

- Brain/CNS/spinal cord
- Cortical regions
- Cerebellum
- Brainstem
- Basal ganglia
- Olfactory bulb
- Thalamus
- Hypothalamus
- Pituitary
- Thyroid
- Upper airways
- Liver
- Adrenals
- Ovaries
- Uterus
- Prostate
- Testes

Locations of CB2 Receptors

- Lymphatic system
- Immune system
- Spleen
- Thymus
- Tonsils
- Blood
- Skin

Locations of CB1 and CB2 Receptors

- Eye
- Stomach
- Heart
- Pancreas
- Digestive tract
- Bone

HOW CANNABINOIDS ATTACH TO RECEPTORS

Like traditional neurotransmitter system models, cannabinoids and their receptors interact in a lock-and-key pattern. However, endocannabinoid receptor dynamics appear to be more intricate than other known receptor systems. CB1 receptors have at least two binding sites on CB receptors, an orthosteric site where THC primarily binds, and allosteric site where CBD, certain terpenes, and other molecules bind to these receptors. When there is a small amount of CBD or other molecules binding to the allosteric sites, then THC easily occupies the primary binding site. However, the occupation of CBD or other molecules on allosteric receptor sites creates conformational changes in the orthosteric receptor region, reducing THC binding to its orthosteric site of action, and altering the resulting biochemical cascades. This is one of the mechanisms in which CBD modulates the effects of THC, which can affect dosing decisions.

Fast Facts

CBD modulates how easily THC can attach to CB1 receptors, thus reducing psychoactivity and potential negative effects of THC.

A separate receptor dynamic, known as "biased-signaling" operates in the ECS. The term "biased signaling" means that the two different endocannabinoid ligands (AEA and 2-AG) give markedly different cellular responses, even when operating on the same receptor, in the same tissue or tissues.

RETROGRADE INHIBITION

Endocannabinoids are the only neurotransmitters that engage in "retrograde signaling," a form of intracellular communication that inhibits immune response, reduces inflammation, relaxes musculature, lowers blood pressure, dilates bronchial passages, and normalizes overstimulated nerves. Retrograde signaling serves as an inhibitory feedback mechanism that tells other neurotransmitters to be quiet when they are firing too fast.

Fast Facts

The ECS is the only neurotransmitter system that uses "retrograde signaling" as an inhibitory feedback mechanism.

Unlike other receptor systems, information from the ECS can flow backward or "upstream" from traditional nerve pathways. This is one of the ways the system's functions protect the nervous system from hyperactivity and excitotoxicity. In traumatic brain injury, increasing in vitro and in vivo data suggest that endocannabinoids have neuroprotective effects through this process of retrograde inhibition. Human and animal models are indicating that when cannabinoids are administered within 4 hours of trauma, they appear to curtail glutamate toxicity and reduce neuronal damage. More research is needed to demonstrate this conclusively.

Fast Facts

Retrograde inhibition quiets overstimulated neurons that cause seizures in illnesses such as epilepsy.

Retrograde inhibition also works on pain pathways in a similar manner. When pain signals are extreme or overwhelming, retrograde inhibition uses cannabinoids to slow or reduce the impulses coming from injury.

> *Research suggests that when cannabinoids are administered within 4 hours of trauma, they appear to curtail glutamate toxicity and reduce neuronal damage.*

Bibliography

Biernacki, M., & Skrzydlewska, E. (2016). Metabolism of endocannabinoids. *Postępy Higieny i Medycyny Doświadczalnej, 70*(0), 830–843.

Colizzi, M., McGuire, P., Pertwee, R. G., & Bhattacharyya, S. (2016). Effect of cannabis on glutamate signaling in the brain: A systematic review of human and animal evidence. *Neuroscience & Biobehavioral Reviews, 64*, 359–381. doi:10.1016/j.neubiorev.2016.03.010

Cowen, P. J., & Browning, M. (2015). What has serotonin to do with depression? *World Psychiatry, 14*(2), 158–160. doi:10.1002/wps.20229

Efrati, I. (2017, May 15). Israel eases restrictions on medical marijuana use and possession. *HAARETZ*. Retrieved from https://www.haaretz.com/israel-news/israel-eases-limits-on-medical-marijuana-1.5472126

Gaoni, Y., & Mechoulam, R. (1964). Isolation, structure, and partial synthesis of an active constituent of hashish. *Journal of the American Chemical Society, 86*(8), 1646–1647. doi:10.1021/ja01062a046

Glass, M., Dragunow, M., & Faull, R. L. (1997). Cannabinoid receptors in the human brain: A detailed anatomical and quantitative autoradiographic study in the fetal, neonatal and adult human brain. *Neuroscience, 77*(2), 299–318. doi:10.1016/s0306-4522(96)00428-9

Gonsiorek, W., Lunn, C., Fan, X., Narula, S., Lundell, D., & Hipkin, R. W. (2000). Endocannabinoid 2-arachidonyl glycerol is a full agonist through human type 2 cannabinoid receptor: Antagonism by anandamide. *Molecular Pharmacology, 57*, 1045–1050.

Guindon, J., & Hohmann, A. G. (2009). The endocannabinoid system and pain. *CNS & Neurological Disorders Drug Targets, 8*(6), 403–421. doi:10.2174/187152709789824660

Hanuš, L. O. (2007). Discovery and isolation of anandamide and other endocannabinoids. *Chemistry & Biodiversity, 4*(8), 1828–1841. doi:10.1002/cbdv.200790154

Herkenham, M., Lynn, A. B., Little, M. D., Johnson, M. R., Melvin, L. S., de Costa, B. R., & Rice, K. C. (1990). Cannabinoid receptor localization in brain. *Proceedings of the National Academy of Sciences of the United States of America, 87*(5), 1932–1936. doi:10.1073/pnas.87.5.1932

Howlett, A. C., Barth, F., Bonner, T. I., Cabral, G., Casellas, P., Devane, W. A., … Pertwee, R. G. (2002). International union of pharmacology. XXVII. Classification of cannabinoid receptors. *Pharmacological Reviews, 54*(2), 161–202.

Howlett, A. C., Blume, L. C., & Dalton, G. D. (2010). CB1 cannabinoid receptors and their associated proteins. *Current Medicinal Chemistry, 17*(14), 1382–1393. doi:10.2174/092986710790980023

Howlett, A. C., Reggio, P. H., Childers, S. R., Hampson, R. E., Ulloa, N. M., & Deutsch, D. G. (2011). Endocannabinoid tone versus constitutive activity of cannabinoid receptors. *British Journal of Pharmacology, 163*(7), 1329–1343. doi:10.1111/j.1476-5381.2011.01364.x

Ibsen, M. S., Connor, M., & Glass, M. (2017). Cannabinoid CB1 and CB2 receptor signaling and bias. *Cannabis and Cannabinoid Research, 2*(1), 48–60. doi:10.1089/can.2016.0037

Inciardi, J. A. (1992). *The war on drugs II.* Mountain View, CA: Mayfield Publishing Company.

Johnson, M., Devane, W., Howlett, A., Melvin, L., & Milne, G. (1988). Structural studies leading to the discovery of a cannabinoid binding site. *NIDA Research Monograph, 90,* 129–135.

Konta, B., & Frank, W. (2008). The treatment of Parkinson's disease with dopamine agonists. *GMS Health Technology Assessment, 4,* Doc05.

Li, S., Wang, L., Liu, M., Jiang, S. K., Zhang, M., Tian, Z. L., … Guan, D. W. (2016). Cannabinoid CB2 receptors are involved in the regulation of fibrogenesis during skin wound repair in mice. *Molecular Medicine Reports, 13*(4), 3441–3450. doi:10.3892/mmr.2016.4961

Lim, G., Sung, B., Ji, R. R., & Mao, J. (2003). Upregulation of spinal cannabinoid-1-receptors following nerve injury enhances the effects of Win 55,212-2 on neuropathic pain behaviors in rats. *Pain, 105*(1–2), 275–283. doi:10.1016/s0304-3959(03)00242-2

Lipsy, R. J., Fennerty, B., & Fagan, T. C. (1990). Clinical review of histamine2 receptor antagonists. *Archives of Internal Medicine, 150*(4), 745–751.

Liu, J., Wang, L., Harvey-White, J., Osei-Hyiaman, D., Razdan, R., Gong, Q., … Kunos, G. (2006). A biosynthetic pathway for anandamide. *PNAS, 103*(36), 13345–13350. doi:10.1073/pnas.0601832103

Lu, H. C., & Mackie, K. (2015). An introduction to the endogenous cannabinoid system. *Biological Psychiatry, 79*(7), 516–525. doi:10.1016/j.biopsych.2015.07.028

Luk, T., Jin, W., Zvonok, A., et al. (2004). Identification of a potent and highly efficacious, yet slowly desensitizing CB1 cannabinoid receptor agonist. *British Journal of Pharmacology, 142,* 495–500. doi:10.1038/sj.bjp.0705792

Mackie, K. (2005). Distribution of cannabinoid receptors in the central and peripheral nervous system. *Handbook of Experimental Pharmacology,* (168), 299–325.

Mackie, K., Devane, W. A., & Hille, B. (1993). Anandamide, an endogenous cannabinoid, inhibits calcium currents as a partial agonist in N18 neuroblastoma cells. *Molecular Pharmacology, 44,* 498–503.

Malfitano, A. M., Basu, S., Maresz, K., Bifulco, M., & Dittel, B. N. (2014). What we know and do not know about the cannabinoid receptor 2 (CB2). *Seminars in Immunology, 26*(5), 369–379. doi:10.1016/j.smim.2014.04.002

McPartland, J. M. (2008). The endocannabinoid system: An osteopathic perspective. *The Journal of the American Osteopathic Association, 108*(10), 586–600. doi:10.7556/jaoa.2008.108.10.586

McPartland, J. M., Matias, I., Di Marzo, V., & Glass, M. (2006). Evolutionary origins of the endocannabinoid system. *Gene, 370*, 64–74. doi:10.1016/j.gene.2005.11.004

Mechoulam, R., Hanuš, L. O., Pertwee, R., & Howlett, A. C. (2014). Early phytocannabinoid chemistry to endocannabinoids and beyond. *Nature Reviews Neuroscience, 15*(11), 757–764. doi:10.1038/nrn3811

Mechoulam, R., Panikashvili, D., & Shohami, E. (2002). Cannabinoids and brain injury: Therapeutic implications. *Trends in Molecular Medicine, 8*(2), 58–61. doi:10.1016/S1471-4914(02)02276-1

Mechoulam, R., & Shohami, E. (2007). Endocannabinoids and traumatic brain injury. *Molecular Neurobiology, 36*(1), 68–74. doi:10.1007/s12035-007-8008-6

Melamede, R. (2010). Endocannabinoids: Multi-scaled, global homeostatic regulators of cells and society. In A. Minai, D. Braha, & Y. Bar-Yam (Eds.), *Unifying themes in complex systems*. Berlin, Germany: Springer.

Pacher, P., Bátkai, S., & Kunos, G. (2006). The endocannabinoid system as an emerging target of pharmacotherapy. *Pharmacological Reviews, 58*(3), 389–462. doi:10.1124/pr.58.3.2

Pacher, P., & Kunos, G. (2013). Modulating the endocannabinoid system in human health and disease–successes and failures. *The FEBS Journal, 280*(9), 1918–1943. doi:10.1111/febs.12260

Panikashvili, D., Simeonidou, C., Ben-Shabat, S., Hanus, L., Breuer, A., Mechoulam, R., & Shohami, E. (2001). An endogenous cannabinoid (2-AG) is neuroprotective after brain injury. *Nature, 413*(6855), 527–531. doi:10.1038/35097089

Pertwee, R. G. (2008). The diverse CB1 and CB2 receptor pharmacology of three plant cannabinoids: Δ9-tetrahydrocannabinol, cannabidiol and Δ9-tetrahydrocannabivarin. *British Journal of Pharmacology, 153*(2), 199–215. doi:10.1038/sj.bjp.0707442

Sidibeh, C. O., Pereira, M. J., Lau Börjesson, J., Kamble, P. G., Skrtic, S., Katsogiannos, P., … Eriksson, J. W. (2017). Role of cannabinoid receptor 1 in human adipose tissue for lipolysis regulation and insulin resistance. *Endocrine, 55*(3), 839–852. doi:10.1007/s12020-016-1172-6

III

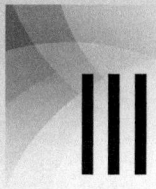

Cannabinoids

6

Cannabinoids and Terpenes

This chapter discusses endogenous and exogenous cannabinoids and the mechanisms through which they interact with the vast network of receptors in the endocannabinoid system (ECS). It also discusses some of the other cannabinoids and terpenes naturally occurring in cannabis and the differences between treating with botanical medicines versus single molecule compounds.

In this chapter, you will learn how to:

- Describe the major and minor cannabinoids found in cannabis.
- Understand how cannabinoids and terpenes affect the ECS.
- Discuss how the entourage effect enhances the medicinal effects of cannabinoids.

MAJOR CANNABINOIDS

Tetrahydrocannabinol (THC) and cannabidiol (CBD) are the major cannabinoids produced by the cannabis plant. These cannabinoids mirror endogenous cannabinoids produced by the body. THC is a mirror image of the endocannabinoid anandamide (AEA), and CBD mirrors 2-arachidonoylglycerol (2-AG).

Tetrahydrocannabinol

THC is the most recognized cannabinoid and is the primary psychoactive compound in cannabis (Figure 6.1). It has been found to be a neuroprotective with analgesic effects.

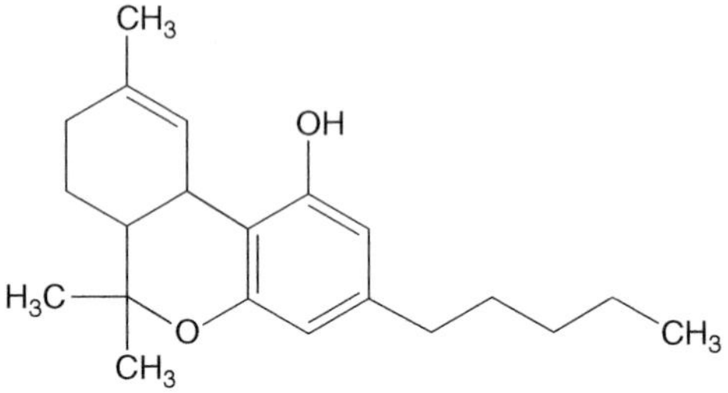

Figure 6.1 Tetrahydrocannabinol (THC) molecule.

THC Properties

- Psychoactive and euphoric effects
- Primarily binds with CB1 receptors
- Treats symptoms of conditions such as:
  - Anxiety
  - Glaucoma
  - Insomnia
  - Muscle spasticity
  - Nausea
  - Appetite
  - Pain

Fast Facts

THC is considered to be a neuroprotective while most illicit drugs are considered to be neurotoxic.

CANNABIDIOL

CBD has been attributed with many medical benefits and has resulted in new hybrid cannabis strains being created to increase the CBD content (Figure 6.2). It has recently been approved by the Food and Drug Administration (FDA) to treat rare and difficult-to-treat forms of epilepsy. CBD can be extracted from industrial hemp, which was legalized in 2018 with the passing of the Farm Bill.

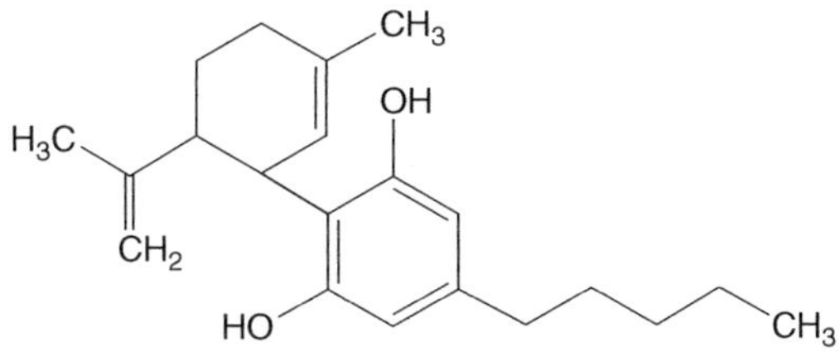

Figure 6.2 Cannabidiol molecule.

CBD Properties

- No psychoactive effect
- Primarily binds with CB2 receptors
- Interferes with THC binding, thus reducing psychoactive effects
- Treats symptoms of conditions such as:
  - Anxiety
  - Seizures
  - Inflammation
  - Depression
  - Migraines
  - Inflammatory bowel disease
  - Pain

Fast Facts

CBD has been found to indirectly help with sleep by easing anxiety symptoms.

MINOR CANNABINOIDS

The two most prevalent cannabinoids are THC and CBD. However, the cannabis plant contains over 600 chemical compounds, and more are discovered each year. Additional cannabinoids are referred to as minor cannabinoids, which are found in smaller quantities in the plant. Of the 113 cannabinoids produced by the plant, only a handful are produced in any significant quantity.

> **Fast Facts**
>
> *The name "minor cannabinoid" is somewhat deceiving: It is not that their power is minor, but they occur in smaller quantities.*

Common Minor Cannabinoids

- Tetrahydrocannabivarin (THCV)
- Cannabinol (CBN)
- Tetrahydrocannabinolic acid (THCA)
- Cannabigerol (CBG)
- Cannabichromene (CBC)
- Cannabidiolic acid (CBDA)
- Cannabidivarin (CBDV)

Cannabigerol

CBG (Figure 6.3) is the third most prevalent cannabinoid after THC and CBD and is more commonly found in hemp varieties than cannabis drug varieties. CBG is analgesic and nonpsychoactive and has been shown to be effective in treating inflammatory bowel disease (IBD) in animal models. Its antiseptic and antibiotic properties are effective in fighting high-resistance staph infections, including MRSA.

- Bone stimulant
- Antibacterial
- Anti-inflammatory
- Antifungal
- Lowers blood pressure
- Inhibits tumor growth

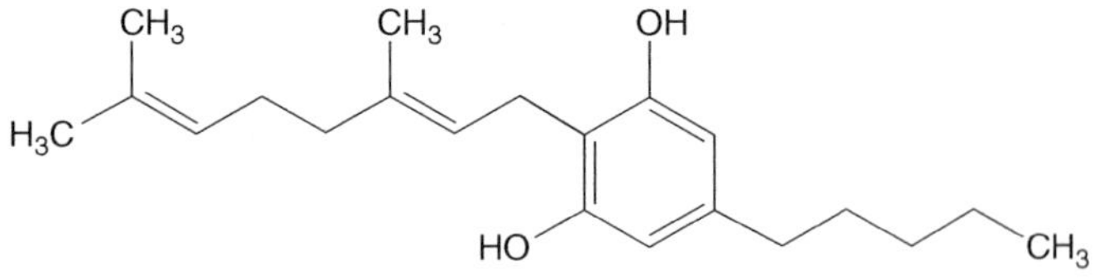

Figure 6.3 Cannabigerol molecule.

Fast Facts

CBG has been found to decrease inflammation associated with IBD in studies involving mice.

Cannabichromene

CBC is rare and produced early in the plant's flowering cycle. It is antibiotic and antifungal, two properties that may protect the plant in its early life. Like many cannabinoids, it is also anti-inflammatory and analgesic and may have some antidepressant effects as well.

- Bone stimulant
- Antibacterial
- Anti-inflammatory
- Antifungal
- Lowers blood pressure
- Relaxes veins

Cannabinol

CBN is not produced by plants, but it is a THC breakdown product that occurs after the oils have dried out (Figure 6.4). It is not psychoactive but does cause sedation when combined with THC, and it has some antiseizure, antibacterial, and analgesic activities, demonstrating that even poorly stored cannabis might have some limited medicinal value. CBN reportedly has three times the affinity for the CB2 receptor than the CB1 receptor, which is why it is believed to have a greater effect on the immune system than the nervous system.

- Relieves spasms
- Pain reliever
- Sleep aid
- Anti-inflammatory
- Antioxidant
- Decreases seizures

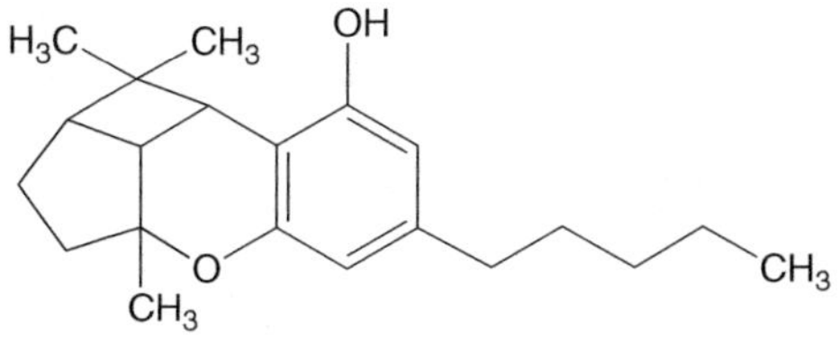

Figure 6.4 Cannabicyclol molecule.

Tetrahydrocannabivarinic

THCV (Figure 6.5) is the bioactive neutral form of tetrahydrocannabivarinic acid or THCVA (Figure 6.6), a propyl form of THC. There is no consensus about whether THCV is psychoactive or merely modulates the psychoactivity of THC. Older research considers THCV to have about 25% of the potency of THC, but more contemporary researh claims that THCV produces no psychoactivity by itself. THCV has analgesic, anti-inflammatory, and anticonvulsant effects—and may encourage weight loss and increased energy expenditure.

- Decreases seizures
- Decreases appetite
- Increases energy expenditure
- Bone stimulant
- Analgesic
- Anti-inflammatory

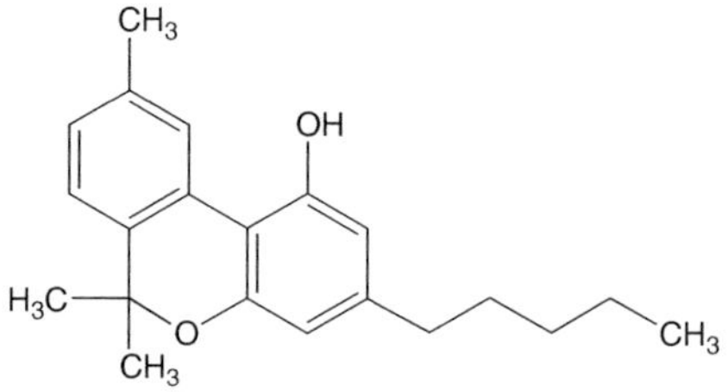

Figure 6.5 Cannabinol molecule.

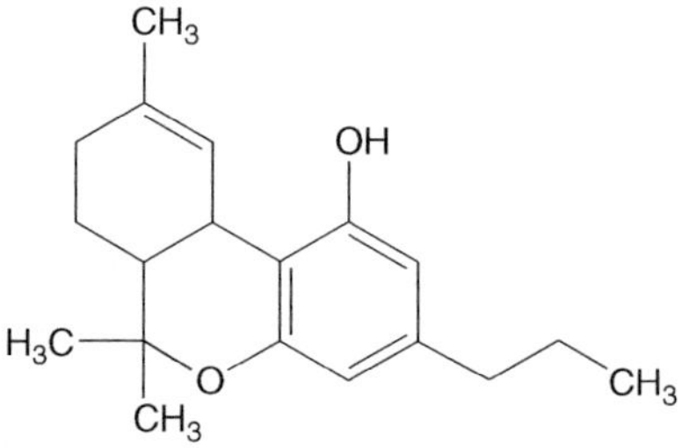

Figure 6.6 Tetrahydrocannabivarin molecule.

Fast Facts

THCV has been found to be an appetite suppressant and can help reduce body weight. It is currently being studied as a treatment for type 2 diabetes.

Figure 6.7 presents a guide for the psychoactive and nonpsychoactive effects of cannabinoids.

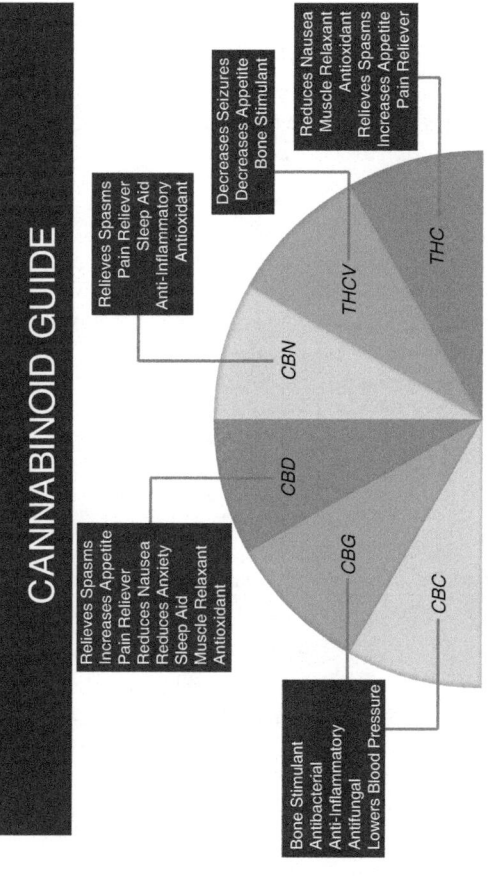

Figure 6.7 Cannabinoid guide.
Source: Medical Marijuana 411. Copyright 2020

TERPENES

Terpenoids (terpenes) represent the largest and most diverse class of chemicals among the myriad compounds produced by plants. Terpenes are powerful odor molecules that are found primarily in the plant's trichomes. Thanks to terpenes, cannabis has such an enduring pungency.

> **Fast Facts**
>
> *It is commonly assumed that THC and CBD cause the powerful aroma of cannabis, but THC and CBD are odorless. The strong aroma of cannabis flower comes from the odor of the terpenes.*

Many plants make terpenes as part of their defense systems. Cannabis has about 200, the most common of which are also key components in lemon, pepper, lavender, hops, and pine. Of these natural compounds, several terpenes are under clinical trials. The most common terpenes found in cannabis are alpha-pinene, linalool, mycrene, limonene, terpineol, beta-caryophyllene, and geraniol. These terpenes are being studied for their anti-inflammatory, analgesic, and sedative effects.

> **Fast Facts**
>
> *You can find terpenes in most plants and foods.*

The terms *indica* and *sativa* are used throughout this book since they are part of the common lexicon, but they are not reliable indicators of the stimulating or sedative qualities of one particular strain. The strength and combination of terpenes are better guides as to how a strain will affect a patient's mood.

Overview of Terpenes

- Terpenes are the most common plant chemicals found in nature—over 30,000 have been identified.
- Cannabis produces more than 200 different terpenes.
- Plants use terpenes to protect themselves from disease, animals, and insects, and even other more invasive plants.

- Initial studies indicate terpenes must exist in a concentration of 0.05% or more of plant material for therapeutic impact.
- Cannabinoids may increase the ability of terpenes to cross the blood–brain barrier.

Table 6.1 describes the odors, medical uses, and benefits of common terpenes.

Table 6.1

Terpenes Chart

Terpene	Smells Like	Medical Use and Benefit
Limonene	Strong citrus—the sour/sharp smell in the rinds of citrus fruits and other flowers. Prevalent in cannabis	Works as an antidepressant and can cause breast cancer cells to commit suicide. It has been used clinically to dissolve gallstones, improve mood, and relieve heartburn and gastrointestinal reflux.
Myrcene	Hops, mango—the "green" musky odor found in bay, thyme, mango, and hops. Prevalent in most types of cannabis	Works as a sedative, muscle relaxant, hypnotic, analgesic, and anti-inflammatory. Also potentiates the effects of THC.
Pinene	Strong pine—most commonly occurring terpenoid	Works as an anti-inflammatory and a bronchodilator. It is potentially helpful for asthma and promotes alertness and memory retention by inhibiting the breakdown of acetylcholinesterase, a neurotransmitter in the brain that stimulates these cognitive effects.
Ocimene	Fruity, floral, and some say "wet cloth" smell	Exhibits anti-inflammatory effects in white blood cells and antifungal effects with the human-specific *Candida* species—has also been effective in fighting the SARS virus. Frequently used in perfumes for its pleasant odor.

(continued)

Table 6.1

Terpenes Chart (*continued*)

Terpene	Smells Like	Medical Use and Benefit
Linalool	Lavender, floral	Antianxiety and stress reducing. A powerful anticonvulsant that also amplifies serotonin-receptor transmission, thus serving as an antidepressant. Found to be a calming sedative and good for sleep.
Beta-caryophyllene	Peppery, clove—found in the background of black pepper, oregano, and clove	Gastroprotective, good for certain ulcers, and shows great promise as a therapeutic compound for inflammatory conditions and autoimmune disorders. Can be used as a dietary supplement with strong anti-inflammatory analgesic effects and has low attributable psychoactivity.
Terpinolene	Pine, sweet herbal, anise, and lime—primarily isolated from trees, present in high amounts in turpentine	Unlike other terpenes, does not have analgesic or anti-inflammatory effects. Works as an antibacterial agent, increases antioxidant capacity levels in white blood cells, and has shown anticancer effects in rat brain cells and anti-insomnia effects in mouse brain cells. Also effective in fighting glial cell cancer and leukemia.
α Humulene	Hoppy, earthy—responsible for an IPA's signature hoppy aroma	Anti-inflammatory, also acts as an appetite suppressant. Most prevalent in hops, where it derives its name, and often found along with beta-caryophyllene. Responsible for the "hoppy" smell of strong beers such as an IPA.

(*continued*)

Table 6.1

Terpenes Chart (continued)

Terpene	Smells Like	Medical Use and Benefit
Nerolidol	Floral, citrus, and some say "fresh bark" smell	Works as a sedative with potent antifungal and antimalarial activity. Further effective in delivering drugs through the skin, and may be a toxin against harmful protozoa such as malaria and leishmaniasis. Low levels are present in orange and other citrus peels.

IPA, India pale ale; THC, tetrahydrocannabinol.

THE ENTOURAGE EFFECT

The medicinal effect of these terpenes and cannabinoids is amplified when they are all used together. This complicated interplay of chemicals is known as the "entourage effect." Put simply: The sum of cannabis' chemical parts is greater than any one of its individual components.

This also explains how cannabis has bedeviled pharmaceutical companies in their attempts to isolate single molecule medicines, such as dronabinol, a synthetic THC approved by the FDA in 1985. Dronabinol is poorly tolerated by patients who report more unpleasant levels of sedation and dysphoria than produced from a whole plant of cannabis. Even though the U.S. government fast-tracked dronabinol's development and placed it in Schedule III to encourage use, patients did not like it and it has never lived up to its promise.

Fast Facts

CBD can help mitigate the negative side effects of THC such as anxiety, irritability, and short-term memory loss.

Another benefit of the entourage effect is that secondary compounds can reduce the negative effects of THC. For example, strains containing high levels of CBD magnify the pain-relieving properties of THC, at the same time reducing anxiety, irritability, and short-term memory loss.

(A) CBD Dominant

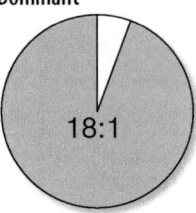

Nonpsychoactive. For novice cannabis users or people who do not want to get high. Some patients find CBD-dominant medicine helpful in anxiety, depression, psychosis, and other mood disorders.

(B) CBD Bridge

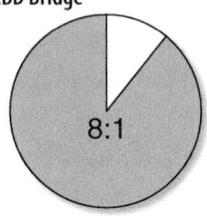

Nonpsychoactive. Some patients find mid-range CBD:THC ratios helpful in spasms, convulsions, tremors, endocrine disorders, metabolic syndrome, and overall wellness.

(C) CBD Harmony

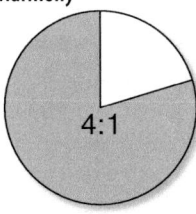

Borderline psychoactive. For patients who have some tolerance for THC. Some patients find mid-range ratios helpful in pain relief, immune support, and other health benefits.

(D) CBD Synergy

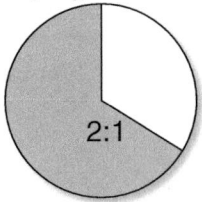

Psychoactive in larger doses. For patients who have some tolerance to THC. Some patients find balanced ratios helpful in chronic pain, gastrointestinal issues, and stress relief.

(E) CBD Balance

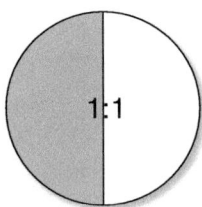

Psychoactive. For patients who can tolerate THC. Some patients find a balanced ratio helpful in neuropathic pain, rheumatism, and overall mood enhancement.

Figure 6.8 Finding your CBD:THC ratio

BOTANICAL VERSUS SINGLE MOLECULE COMPOUNDS

Botanical medicines behave differently than conventional single molecule drugs. In fact, the FDA places botanical drugs in a separate regulatory class. In its 2004 white paper on this topic, the FDA discusses these differences. "Non-clinical data may be appropriate to help establish safe doses (for botanicals) and to determine ways to better monitor potential toxicities in humans." In 2016, the FDA reiterated this position.

Why cannabis is subjected to the same clinical trials as other single pharmaceutical compounds is much debated. The U.S. government attempts to address this discrepancy by classifying cannabis as a Schedule I substance that has a high potential for abuse with no medical value. If it were to be descheduled, cannabinoid medicines could be categorized as botanical drugs, and their regulation could fall under this guidance. In other words, botanicals are living organisms, and it is more difficult to subject botanical medicines to the same sorts of clinical studies as single molecule substances.

Bibliography

Appendino, G., Gibbons, S., Glana, A., Pagani, A., Grassi, G., Stavri, M., … Rahman, M. M. (2008). Antibacterial cannabinoids from cannabis sativa: A structure–activity study. *Journal of Natural Products, 71*(8), 1427–1430. doi:10.1021/np8002673

Borrelli, F., Fasolino, I., Romano, B., Capasso, R., Maiello, F., Coppola, D., … Izzo, A. A. (2013). Beneficial effect of the non-psychotropic plant cannabinoid cannabigerol on experimental inflammatory bowel disease. *Biochemical Pharmacology, 85*(9), 1306–1316. doi:10.1016/j.bcp.2013.01.017

Brennesien, R. (2007). Chemistry and analysis of phytocannabinoids and other cannabis constituents. In M. ElSohly (Ed.), *Marijuana and the cannabinoids* (pp. 17–49). Totowa, NJ: Humana Press Inc.

Deyo, R., & Musty, R. (2003). A cannabichromene (CBC) extract alters behavioral despair on the mouse tail suspension test of depression. In *13th Symposium on the Cannabinoids* (p. 146). Cornwall, ON: International Cannabinoid Research Society.

dos Santos, R., Hallak, J., Leite, J., Zuardi, A. W., & Crippa, J. A. (2015). Phytocannabinoids and epilepsy. *Journal of Clinical Pharmacy and Therapeutics, 40*(2), 135–143. doi:10.1111/jcpt.12235

ElSohly, H., Turner, C., Clark, A., & ElSohly, M. (1982). Synthesis and antimicrobial activities of certain cannabichromene and cannabigerol related compounds. *Journal of Pharmaceutical Sciences, 71*(12), 1319–1323. doi:10.1002/jps.2600711204

McPartland, J., & Russo, E. (2001). Cannabis and cannabis extracts. *Journal of Cannabis Therapeutics, 1*(3–4), 103–132.

Russo, E. (2011). Taming THC: Potential cannabis synergy and phytocannabinoid-terpenoid entourage effects. *British Journal of Pharmacology, 163*(7), 1344–1364. doi:10.1111/j.1476-5381.2011.01238.x

Tholl, D. (2015). Biosynthesis and biological functions of terpenoids in plants. *Advances in Biochemical Engineering/Biotechnology, 148*, 63–106. doi:10.1007/10_2014_295

US Department of Health and Human Services, Food and Drug Administration Center for Drug Evaluation and Research. (2016). *Guidance for industry: Botanical drug products*. Washington, DC: US Government Publishing Office.

Whiteley, N. (2016). *Chronic relief: A guide to cannabis for the terminally & chronically ill*. Austin, TX: Alivio LLC.

7

Synthetic Cannabinoid Pharmaceuticals

This chapter is an overview listing the research, intended use, and availability of synthetic Food and Drug Administration (FDA)–approved cannabinoid medications in the United States today. It is a resource for nurses who assist patients who are currently taking these cannabinoids as part of their prescribed treatment plan.

In this chapter, you will learn how to:

- Identify all current FDA-approved synthetic cannabinoids.
- List common adverse effects and patient-reported reactions to synthetic cannabinoids.
- Understand onset, dosing, and bioavailability of synthetic cannabinoids.

FDA-APPROVED CANNABINOID MEDICATIONS

The FDA has approved four cannabinoid medications to date and is expected to approve a second *Cannabis sativa* extract in 2019.

Current FDA-Approved Medications

- Dronabinol (MarinolD)
- Nabilone (CesametN)
- Dronabinol oral solution (SyndrosD)
- Cannabidiol (EpidiolexC)

The FDA has reviewed several other synthetic cannabinoid drugs in the past decade; however, these were not approved. The most notorious synthetic cannabinoid was rimonabant, an anti-obesity drug that was an inverse agonist of CB1 receptors. This was later withdrawn worldwide in 2008 due to serious and life-threatening psychiatric adverse effects or severe depression, including suicide.

SYNTHETIC CANNABINOID MEDICATION INFORMATION

- There is a high degree of pharmacokinetic variability among patients. Fasting versus administration with food can also cause variability to onset.
- Therapeutic effects last for 24 hours or longer. However, they are usually taken twice daily. The efficacy of an appetite stimulant lasts at least 5 months according to the studies.
- Studies of chemotherapy-induced nausea and vomiting show efficacy. However, it has a slow onset of action, and new antiemetics, 5HT-3 and NK-1 antagonists, seem to be superior. Synthetic cannabinoid pharmaceuticals can be combined with other antiemetics.

Fast Facts

Persons with a personal or strong family history of psychosis, schizophrenia, or panic disorder have a relative contraindication to the use of synthetic cannabinoids.

CONTRAINDICATIONS OF SYNTHETIC CANNABINOID MEDICATIONS

- *Adverse effects can be a particular problem in elderly patients* or persons with a comorbid condition that affects memory or coordination. Synthetic cannabinoids may also lower the seizure threshold.

- Due to lack of safety and efficacy data, synthetic cannabinoids are *not recommended for use in children or adolescents below 18 years of age.* There is suggestive evidence in tissue culture, animal models, and population studies that use of delta-9-tetrahydrocannabinol (THC) in adolescents can have an impact on cognitive functions due to the increased neuroplasticity in this age group.
- Synthetic cannabinoids are a fat-soluble drug, therefore they may be present in the fetus and breast milk. *Pregnancy and breastfeeding are strong relative contraindications.*

DRONABINOL (MARINOL®) CAPSULES

In 1985, the FDA approved the first cannabinoid medication, dronabinol, which was before the ECS was discovered.

Fast Facts

Dronabinol was approved to work as an appetite stimulant in wasting syndromes, and an antiemetic in people receiving chemotherapy.

Dronabinol Facts

- Synthetic analog of delta-9-THC
- Available in 2.5, 5, and 10 mg soft gelatin capsules
- Dose is ingested and goes through a first-pass effect of the liver
- Due to the first-pass effect, only 10% to 20% of the drug reaches the circulation
- Onset of action is 30 to 60 minutes and the peak is 2 to 4 hours

Dronabinol is not bioidentical to organic THC found in *Cannabis sativa*. Unlike THC from plants or genetically modified yeast, which is a partial agonist, dronabinol is a synthetic full agonist of CB1 receptors.

Studies in patients with HIV-associated cachexia show increased body weight, improved mood, and decreased nausea.

Fast Facts

Dronabinol is a pure CB1 full agonist and therefore has several significant adverse effects, including sympathomimetic effects such as tachycardia, hypertension, anxiety, and orthostatic hypotension.

It has a higher potential for abuse and more euphoric and psychoactive effects, so it requires closer physician supervision than other cannabinoid medications.

> **Fast Facts**
>
> *Persons with a history of substance abuse may chew or open the capsules to get more rapid oromucosal absorption and miss the first-pass effect, resulting in euphoria.*

Patients Report

- Dose-related euphoria and elation
- Outbursts of uncontrollable laughter
- Heightened awareness
- Effects can last 4 to 6 hours

Patients usually develop a tolerance to these euphoric side effects within 2 weeks.

Common Adverse Effects

- Short-term memory loss
- Confusion
- Drowsiness
- Reduced coordination

It was originally placed on Schedule II of the Controlled Substances Act (CSA); however, it was rescheduled to Schedule III in 1999 based on clinical experience.

An overdose of dronabinol can result in a temporary episode of several hours of severe agitation, anxiety, dysphoria, and tachycardia. Cannabidiol doses of 200 mg taken oromucosally have been reported to significantly improve these overdose effects in case reports.

NABILONE (CESAMET®) CAPSULES

Also in 1985, the FDA approved another synthetic cannabinoid medication, nabilone.

Nabilone Facts

- Synthetic analog of delta-9-THC
- Available in 1 mg capsules
- The dose is ingested and goes through a first-pass effect of the liver
- Due to the first-pass effect, only 10% to 20% of the drug reaches the circulation
- Onset of action is 30 to 60 minutes and the peak is 2 to 4 hours

Similar to dronabinol, it is not bioidentical to organic THC found in the *C. sativa* plant. It is a full agonist of CB1 receptors, unlike naturally occurring THC, which is a partial agonist.

Fast Facts

FDA documentation of nabilone reveals that studies in patients with HIV-associated cachexia show increased body weight, improved mood, and decreased nausea.

This drug was approved as an antiemetic in people receiving chemotherapy who have failed to respond to conventional medications.

Fast Facts

Nabilone is a synthetic and pure CB1 full agonist, and therefore has several significant adverse effects, including sympathomimetic effects including tachycardia, hypertension, anxiety, and orthostatic hypotension.

Nabilone has more euphoric and psychoactive effects than dronabinol, which may result in a higher potential for abuse. Therefore, it requires close physician supervision, and greater control of dispensing than the other cannabinoid medications.

Patients Report

- Dose-related euphoria and elation
- Outbursts of uncontrollable laughter
- Heightened awareness
- Effects can last up to 4 to 6 hours

Patients usually develop a tolerance to these euphoric side effects within 2 weeks.

Common Adverse Effects

- Short-term memory loss
- Confusion
- Drowsiness
- Reduced coordination

Persons with a history of substance abuse may chew or open the capsules to get more rapid oromucosal absorption and miss the first-pass effect, resulting in euphoria. Due to the heightened risk of euphoria and abuse, it is on Schedule II of the CSA.

An overdose of nabilone can result in a temporary episode of several hours of severe agitation, dysphoria, and tachycardia.

Fast Facts

Cannabidiol dose of 200 mg taken oromucosally has been reported to significantly improve these overdose effects in many case reports.

DRONABINOL ORAL SOLUTION (SYNDROS®)

A new formulation of dronabinol, in an oral solution, was approved by the FDA in 2016. This allows for titration and stricter control of the dose than the older capsules with a limited choice of doses. This superior control of dosing and titration leads to an improved adverse effect profile compared with the older capsules.

Dronabinol Oral Solution Facts

- Synthetic analog of delta-9-THC
- Available in an orally swallowed formulation of 5 mg/mL
- The dose is ingested and goes through a first-pass effect of the liver
- Due to the first-pass effect, only 10% to 20% of the drug reaches the circulation
- Onset of action is 30 to 60 minutes and the peak is 2 to 4 hours

It is synthetic and is not bioidentical to organic THC found in the *C. sativa* plant. Unlike THC from plants, or genetically modified yeast, which is a partial agonist, dronabinol is a full agonist of CB1 receptors.

This drug was approved to work as an appetite stimulant in wasting syndromes, and an as antiemetic in people receiving chemotherapy. Studies in patients with HIV-associated cachexia show increased body weight, improved mood, and decreased nausea.

Fast Facts

Dronabinol's efficacy as an appetite stimulant lasts at least 5 months according to the studies.

Unlike the other drug formulations already discussed, it can easily be used oromucosally, instead of being ingested, to obtain much more rapid onset of action, with euphoric and other psychoactive effects compared with ingestion.

Patients Report

- Dose-related euphoria and elation
- Outbursts of uncontrollable laughter
- Heightened awareness
- Effects can last 4 to 6 hours

Patients usually develop a tolerance to these euphoric side effects within 2 weeks.

Common Adverse Effects

- Short-term memory loss
- Confusion
- Drowsiness
- Reduced coordination

Fast Facts

Persons with a history of substance abuse may not swallow the liquid but instead keep it under their tongue to get more rapid oromucosal absorption and miss the first-pass effect, resulting in rapid onset of euphoria.

Bibliography

Bhattacharyya, S., Morrison, P. D., Fusar-Poli, P., Martin-Santos, R., Borgwardt, S., Winton-Brown, T., ... McGuire, P. K. (2010). Opposite effects of delta-9-tetrahydrocannabinol and cannabidiol on human brain function and psychopathology. *Neuropsychopharmacology, 35*(3), 764–774. doi:10.1038/npp.2009.184

Egan, A. (2007). *NDA 21-888 Zimutli (rimonabant) Tablets, 20mg Sanofi Aventis Advisory Committee—June 13, 2007* (p. 88). *Food and Drug Administration Dronabinol fact sheet.*

Food and Drug Administration dronabinol fact sheet. Rev 08/2017

Food and Drug Administration dronabinol oral solution. Rev 05/2017

Food and Drug Administration nabilone fact sheet. Rev 05/2006

Gorter, R. W. (1999). Cancer cachexia and cannabinoids. *Forsch Komplementarmed, 6*(Suppl. 3), 21–22. doi:10.1159/000057152

May, M. B., & Glode, A. E. (2016). Dronabinol for chemotherapy-induced nausea and vomiting unresponsive to antiemetics. *Cancer Management and Research, 8,* 49–55. doi:10.2147/CMAR.S81425

Ware, M. A., Daeninck, P., & Maida, V. (2008). A review of nabilone in the treatment of chemotherapy-induced nausea and vomiting. *Therapeutics and Clinical Risk Management, 4*(1), 99–107. doi:10.2147/tcrm.s1132

8

Isolate Cannabinoid Pharmaceuticals

This chapter is an overview listing the research, intended use, and availability of isolate Food and Drug Administration (FDA)–approved cannabinoid medications in the United States today. It is a resource for nurses who assist patients who are currently taking these cannabinoids as part of their prescribed treatment plan.

In this chapter, you will learn how to:

- Identify all current FDA-approved isolate cannabinoids.
- Summarize the formulation of plant extract cannabinoid medications.
- List the differences between pharmaceutical grade and non–FDA-approved cannabinoid medications.

CANNABIDIOL (EPIDIOLEX®)

Epidiolex is a 99% cannabidiol (CBD) isolate extracted from *Cannabis sativa* approved by the FDA in 2018. As a pure isolate of CBD, it does not have the combined entourage effect from minor cannabinoids and terpenes. Cannabidiol increases the amount of naturally occurring anandamide (AEA) available at the CB1 and CB2 receptors by blocking metabolic enzymes and transport proteins.

Cannabidiol Facts

- Oral solution with an oral syringe for intraoral administration
- Absorbed rapidly via the intraoral route directly into the circulation
- Any drug that may be ingested goes through the first-pass effect of the liver, which metabolizes about 85% of the cannabidiol to inactive metabolites
- Onset of action is approximately 15 minutes with peak concentrations at 45 to 120 minutes

Plant extract administered oromucosally reaches maximum plasma levels at 60 minutes. Additionally, some of the CBD may be ingested and undergo hepatic first-pass metabolism. The doses used for pediatric intractable seizures are much higher, 5 to 25 mg/kg, than the doses used to treat most other conditions.

It has received the Rare Pediatric Disease and Orphan Drug Designations from the FDA for treatment of Dravet and Lennox–Gastaut syndromes (LGS). Trials are underway for tuberous sclerosis (TS) and infantile spasm (IS).

Common Adverse Effects

- Somnolence
- Fatigue
- Increased or decreased appetite

It has a low risk of abuse and dependency due to a balancing effect of CBD at the CB1 receptor, which significantly decreases euphoric and psychoactive effects.

Fast Facts

Even though cannabis sativa is a Schedule I drug, this isolated extract of cannabis is listed as a Schedule V drug.

Cannabidiol Extract Research

During this cannabidiol study, 261 patients received at least 3 months of treatment.

Diagnoses included:

- Dravet syndrome
- Myoclonic-absence epilepsy
- Lennox–Gastaut
- Generalized epilepsies
- Other forms of treatment-resistant epilepsy

The median overall seizure frequency reduction:

- 45.1% in all patients
- 62.7% in Dravet syndrome patients
- 71.1% in Lennox–Gastaut syndrome patients

Of all patients, 47% had a ≥50% reduction in seizures. Seizure-freedom at 3 months occurred in 9% of patients and 13% of Dravet syndrome patients.

Adverse Events in ≥10% of Patients

- Somnolence
- Diarrhea
- Fatigue
- Decreased appetite
- Convulsions
- Vomiting

Adverse Events by the Numbers

- Fourteen patients (4%) had an adverse event leading to discontinuation of cannabidiol.
- Thirty-six patients (12%) withdrew primarily due to lack of efficacy.
- About 106 (34%) patients reported serious adverse events
    - Seven deaths occurred, none of which were considered treatment-related.
- Sixteen patients (5%) had serious adverse effects that were considered treatment-related
    - Altered liver enzymes in four patients, all of whom were also on valproate and clobazam; status epilepticus/convulsion; diarrhea; decreased weight; thrombocytopenia; and others

Fast Facts

There are over 150 high-quality research studies completed or in process for various therapeutic effects of CBD, either as an isolate or as whole-plant extracts.

CBD Treatment Studies

- Chronic pain
- Neurodegenerative conditions
- Adult and pediatric epilepsy
- Anxiety
- Tremor
- Graft-versus-host disease
- Psychosis
- Crohn's disease

NABIXIMOLS (SATIVEX®)

Nabiximols is a whole plant extract from two strains of *C. sativa*. It contains an approximate 1:1 ratio of CBD to THC. Since strains of cannabis with a 1:1 ratio of CBD to THC do not generally exist, two different strains were necessary to achieve this goal. One strain is high in CBD and very low in THC. The other strain is low in CBD and high in THC. Cannabis is grown under very strict conditions, and good manufacturing practices are employed to ensure consistency, potency, quality, and lack of contamination from batch to batch.

Nabiximols Facts

- Oromucosal spray
- Absorbed into the circulation from the oromucosal cavity
- Each bottle contains 100 sprays
- Each spray has 2.7 mg of THC and 2.5 mg of CBD
- Also contains small amounts of minor cannabinoids and terpenes
- Onset of action is approximately 15 minutes with peak concentrations at 45 to 120 minutes

Plant extract administered oromucosally compared with inhaled vaporized THC extract has far lower peak plasma concentrations, 5.4 ng/mL versus 118.6 ng/mL, and maximum plasma levels of 60 minutes compared with 17 minutes. THC and CBD are metabolized in the liver. Additionally, some of the THC undergoes hepatic first-pass metabolism to 11-OH-THC, the primary metabolite of THC, and CBD similarly to 7-OH-CBD.

Protein binding of THC is high (approximately 97%). THC and CBD may be stored for as long as four weeks in the fatty tissues from which they are slowly released at subtherapeutic levels back into the bloodstream, then metabolized and excreted via urine and feces.

> **Fast Facts**
>
> *Nabiximols has been approved in over 30 countries as a prescription pharmaceutical since 2010.*

Nabiximols has successfully completed phase 3 trials in the United States and is expected to be approved by the FDA by the end of 2019. This drug has been approved to treat MS spasticity and neuropathic and chronic cancer pain in many countries. Nabiximols is a CB1 and CB2 partial agonist. THC extracts such as nabiximols have several adverse effects at higher doses, usually above 10 mg of THC per dose.

Common Adverse Effects

- Dizziness
- Drowsiness
- Disorientation

Adverse Events in ≥10% of Patients

- Tachycardia
- Hypertension
- Anxiety
- Orthostatic hypotension

The phase 3 studies show that it has a low risk of abuse and dependency due to balancing the effect of CBD at the CB1 receptor, which significantly decreases euphoric and psychoactive effects. Nabiximols may produce undesirable effects such as dizziness and somnolence, which may impair judgment and performance of skilled tasks. Patients should not drive, operate machinery, or engage in any hazardous activity if they are experiencing any significant CNS effects such as dizziness or somnolence. Patients should be aware that nabiximols has been known to cause loss of consciousness in a few cases.

It may interact with alcohol, affecting coordination, concentration, and ability to respond quickly. In general, alcoholic beverages should be avoided while using nabiximols, especially at the beginning of treatment or when changing the dose. Patients should be advised that if they do drink alcohol while using nabiximols, the additive effects may impair their ability to drive or use machinery and may increase the risk of falls.

> **Fast Facts**
>
> *Nabiximols has a risk of increased incidence of falls in patients whose spasticity has been reduced and whose muscle strength is insufficient to maintain posture or gait.*

In addition to an increased risk of falls, the CNS adverse reactions of nabiximols, particularly in elderly patients, could potentially have an impact on various aspects of personal safety, such as with food and hot drink preparation.

> **Fast Facts**
>
> *Care should be taken when combining nabiximols and hypnotics, sedatives, and drugs with potentially sedating effects as there may be an additive effect on sedation and muscle-relaxing effects.*

As with all THC-containing preparations, nabiximols is contraindicated in a patient with any known or suspected history or family history of schizophrenia or other psychotic illness; history of severe personality disorder or other significant psychiatric disorder other than depression associated with their underlying condition.

> **Fast Facts**
>
> *An overdose of nabiximols can result in a temporary episode of several hours of severe agitation, dysphoria, and tachycardia.*

Persons with a history of substance abuse may take more than the recommended dose to experience increased euphoric effects.

CONTRAINDICATIONS OF ISOLATE CANNABINOIDS

Cannabinoid isolates are *not recommended for use in children or adolescents below 18 years of age* due to lack of safety and efficacy data. There is suggestive evidence in tissue culture, animal models, and population studies that use of THC in adolescents can have an impact on cognitive functions due to the increased neuroplasticity in this age group.

Cannabinoid isolates are a fat-soluble drug and therefore may be present in the fetus and breast milk. *Pregnancy and breastfeeding are strong relative contraindications* to the use of cannabinoid medications.

FUTURE CANNABINOID PHARMACEUTICALS

The current and foreseeable trend for FDA-approved cannabinoid pharmaceuticals will be using whole plant extracts that contain naturally occurring versions of various cannabinoids, including THC, CBD, tetrahydrocannabivarin (THCV), and cannabinol (CBN). Plant geneticists are developing new strains of *C. sativa* that have high percentages of these other cannabinoids so that scalable quantities of THCV, CBN, and other minor cannabinoids will be available for pharmaceutical manufacturing. Additional clinical research is needed to determine how each of these cannabinoids can be used in future FDA-approved pharmaceuticals.

Current Cannabinoid Clinical Trials

- Epilepsy
- Autism spectrum disorders
- Neonatal hypoxic-ischemic encephalopathy
- Glioblastoma
- Schizophrenia

Isolate Versus Whole Plant Extract Dosing Curve

The cannabidiol extract is a 99% isolate with essentially no terpenes or minor cannabinoids. The *C. sativa* extract nabiximols is a whole plant extract rich with minor cannabinoids and terpenes. A new study in an animal model shows that isolate-based extracts (monomolecular) are not as effective as whole plant extracts equivalent to milligram doses. Isolates have an inverse U-shaped dose–response curve with a narrow therapeutic window. The addition of the entourage effect from the minor cannabinoids and terpenes moves the dose–response curve to the left, with therapeutic benefits seen at lower doses.

Fast Facts

Whole plant extracts containing major cannabinoids, minor cannabinoids, and terpenes have demonstrated greater therapeutic benefits with lower doses.

FEDERAL FARM BILL (2018) AND ACCESS TO CANNABIDIOL

In December 2018, the U.S. Congress passed the 2018 farm bill with extensive provisions that legalized growing and manufacturing hemp, and transporting and selling of hemp products, including certain hemp-derived products for human consumption throughout the United States. Hemp is defined as cannabis that contains less than 0.3% THC. The 2018 Farm Bill removed all hemp-derived products from the DEA's Schedule I of the CSA and allowed for nonprescription access to hemp-derived cannabinoid extracts, vaporizers, edibles, drinks, hemp flower, and topicals.

Fast Facts

Although hemp-derived CBD is no longer a Schedule I drug, it may still be illegal in your state. Some states have zero tolerance cannabis policies on the books, which include CBD products.

The FDA has now taken over supervision of these products and formulations. It is expected to enforce the manufacturing, quality assurance, consistency, and formulation standards of these products so that they will be in line with the millions of other products overseen by the FDA. Historically, these hemp-derived CBD formulations have not been manufactured with good manufacturing practices. In addition, the labeling has been inconsistent with the actual potency of CBD contained within a majority of the products. FDA supervision is expected to address these previous quality and safety concerns.

Fast Facts

A study published in the Journal of the American Medical Association in 2017 found that nearly 70% of all CBD products sold online are incorrectly labeled and could cause serious harm to consumers.

Safety Concerns of Non–FDA-Approved CBD

- Discrepancies in claimed CBD content
- Inconsistent recommended dosing
- Poor manufacturing practices
- Added chemicals
- Carrier ingredient allergies

People are able to purchase hemp-derived cannabinoid formulations that are high in CBD, and combined with whole plant non-THC cannabinoids that include the entourage components of terpenes and minor cannabinoids. These products generally cost a fraction of the price per dose of the FDA-approved cannabinoid medications, and providers should become familiar with these formulations so that they can advise and educate their patients, and understand dose–response curves, dosing, and routes of administration.

Bibliography

Bolognini, D. (2010). *Pharmacological properties of the phytocannabinoids Δ9-tetrahydrocannabivarin and cannabidiol*. Retrieved from https://www.semanticscholar.org/paper/Pharmacological-properties-of-the-phytocannabinoids-Bolognini/1751b10ef52520f4224c3cb7ada6c0a6e975e86c

Bonn-Miller, M. O., Loflin, M. J. E., Thomas, B. F., Marcu, J. P., Hyke, T., & Vandrey, R. (2017). Labeling accuracy of cannabidiol extracts sold online. *JAMA, 318*(17), 1708–1709. doi:10.1001/jama.2017.11909

Borgelt, L. M., Franson, K. L., Nussbaum, A. M., & Wang, G. S. (2013). The pharmacologic and clinical effects of medical cannabis. *Pharmacotherapy, 33*(2), 195–209. doi:10.1002/phar.1187

Conaway, K. M. (2018). *H.R.2—115th Congress (2017–2018): Agriculture improvement act of 2018.*

Devinsky, O., Thiele, E., Laux, L., Friedman, D., Patel, A., Bluvstein, J., … Marsh, E. (2015). *Efficacy and safety of epidiolex (cannabidiol) in children and young adults with treatment-resistant epilepsy: Update from the Expanded Access Program*. Chicago, IL: American Epilepsy Society.

Food and Drug Administration Epidiolex fact sheet. Rev 2/2018. Retrieved from https://www.accessdata.fda.gov/drugsatfda_docs/label/2018/210365lbl.pdf

Gallily, R., Yekhtin, Z., & Hanuš, L. O. (2015). Overcoming the bell-shaped dose-response of cannabidiol by using cannabis extract enriched in cannabidiol. *Pharmacology & Pharmacy, 6*(02), 75–85. doi:10.4236/pp.2015.62010

McGilveray, I. J. (2005). Pharmacokinetics of cannabinoids. *Pain Research and Management, 10*(Suppl. A), 15A–22A. doi:10.1155/2005/242516

Perucca, E. (2017). Cannabinoids in the treatment of epilepsy: Hard evidence at last? *Journal of Epilepsy Research, 7*(2), 61–76. doi:10.14581/jer.17012

Sativex Oromucosal Spray. Electronic Medicines Compendium. Rev 8/2018. Retrieved from https://www.medicines.org.uk/emc/product/602/smpc

Wade, D. T., Collin, C., Stott, C., & Duncombe, P. (2010). Meta-analysis of the efficacy and safety of Sativex (nabiximols), on spasticity in people with multiple sclerosis. *Multiple Sclerosis, 16*(6), 707–714. doi:10.1177/1352458510367462

IV

Medical Marijuana

9

Medical Marijuana and Bioavailability

This chapter familiarizes you with the many methods of delivering cannabinoids into the bloodstream—inhalation, oral mucosal absorption, edibles, and topicals—plus the advantages and disadvantages of each. Included are written and visual descriptions of all forms of medical cannabis that a patient might encounter in a dispensary, plus the instruments that deliver them. This section also includes guides to onset times, duration of effects, and bioavailability with each method.

In this chapter, you will learn how to:

- Compare the various ways a patient can medicate with medical marijuana.
- Understand the onset times and duration of effects of the most common types of medical marijuana.
- Explain how the bioavailability changes depending on the form of medical marijuana.

MEDICAL MARIJUANA PROGRAMS

As of March 2020, 33 states in the United States had enacted laws creating medical marijuana programs to protect patients who use cannabis for various state-approved medical conditions. Each state has unique rules and regulations regarding this controversial decision to go against federal policy on the legality of cannabis. Without federal guidelines, this has created a wide range of products, types of dispensaries, how to obtain a doctor's recommendation, and quantity of medicine a patient can purchase. When discussing medical marijuana with a patient be aware of how a patient can dose, how much they are allowed to purchase, and where they can purchase medical marijuana. Doctors and nurses cannot prescribe medical marijuana in any state but you can be knowledgeable regarding your state's basic guidelines.

ROLE OF DISPENSARIES

The dispensary is usually the first place patients encounter the full range of products available to them. The experience can be overwhelming (and a little bit thrilling) to new patients. Medical professionals need an understanding of how these institutions function and how widely dispensary experiences can vary.

Fast Facts

Dispensary personnel cannot give medical advice or specific dosing information to treat medical conditions.

Patients likely interact with certified dispensary personnel, otherwise known as "budtenders." Dispensary personnel serve patients but they are not medically trained. State laws allow them to share anecdotal information about products and what other patients have used for treatment but cannot recommend products for medical conditions. In addition, many states do not require state-approved training and licensing for consultants who interact with patients.

What Dispensary Consultants Can Say

- "In my experience…"
- "Patients have said…"
- "Anecdotally I hear…"

What Dispensary Consultants Cannot Say

- "I recommend…"
- "Buy this…"
- "This really works. It is the best for…"

FLOWERS VERSUS CONCENTRATES

Pipes, joints, water pipes, electronic vaporizers as large as blenders or as portable as pens…there are as many ways of delivering cannabis into the system. You should be familiar with the best devices to deliver the precise dose for the desired duration with fewest adverse reactions for patients. This can be a challenge for providers and cannabis-naive patients alike, but this module provides a thorough overview of the various options.

Cannabis Flower

Dried cannabis flowers are the most widely used form of cannabis (Figure 9.1), though this is changing with the advent of concentrates, tinctures, and edibles.

Fast Facts

Patients choosing cannabis flower experience the benefits of all the cannabinoids and terpenes present in the strain.

In the recreational market, cannabis flowers are typically identified by strains, but medical professionals can find more detailed

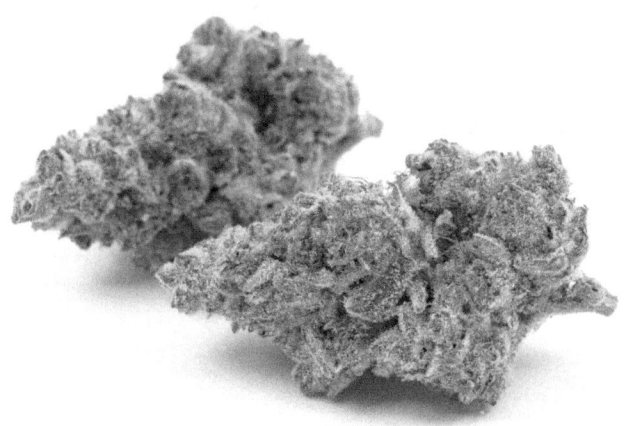

Figure 9.1 Cannabis flower.

information about the cannabinoid and terpene profiles by looking at gas or liquid chromatography lab testing. Though tests vary from lab to lab, they are more reliable guides to effects than strain classification.

> **Fast Facts**
>
> *Cannabis flower may not contain a high enough concentration of cannabinoids needed to treat some conditions.*

Advantages of Cannabis Flower
- Lower cost to patient
- More widely available
- Can be grown at home if legal in the patient's state
- Contains all cannabinoids and terpenes in the strain profile

Disadvantages of Cannabis Flower
- Cannabinoid content may not be high enough for treatment
- Carcinogens and plant material may be inhaled
- Improper storage can lead to mold and plant degradation

Cannabis Concentrates

Dabs, shatter, wax, budder, butane hash oil (BHO), and rosin are all different names for styles of cannabis extracts known as concentrates. Concentrates refer to the oils and terpenes once they are stripped from the plant. Though they come in different forms, all concentrates are many times more powerful than flowers and are used to relieve symptoms of opiate, alcohol, or other drug withdrawals, plus other extreme pain conditions.

> **Fast Facts**
>
> *Concentrates allow patients to take large doses of cannabinoids quickly.*

Concentrates are consumed by vaporization or by "dabbing," a process in which a tiny sesame-size amount of concentrate is placed on a scorching hot surface and inhaled. To give you context for the potency of these concentrates, a powerful strain of cannabis contains 20% tetrahydrocannabinol (THC); a dab can reach 70% or 80% concentration of THC.

Fast Facts

Concentrates require a larger amount of plant matter to manufacture. Patients should choose pesticide-free, lab-tested products to avoid health concerns from unwanted chemicals.

Different Forms of Concentrates

- BHO is the most popular concentrate—it has a gooey, thick, tar-like consistency (Figure 9.2).
- "Budder" or "wax" contains some of the waxy coverings that contain the oils on the plant, which gives them a more opaque and crumbly texture (Figure 9.3).
- "Shatter" resembles a translucent amber candy (Figure 9.4). Though it has a reputation for being the purest and cleanest type of extract, translucence is not a sign of quality. Purity comes down to the way these oils are extracted.

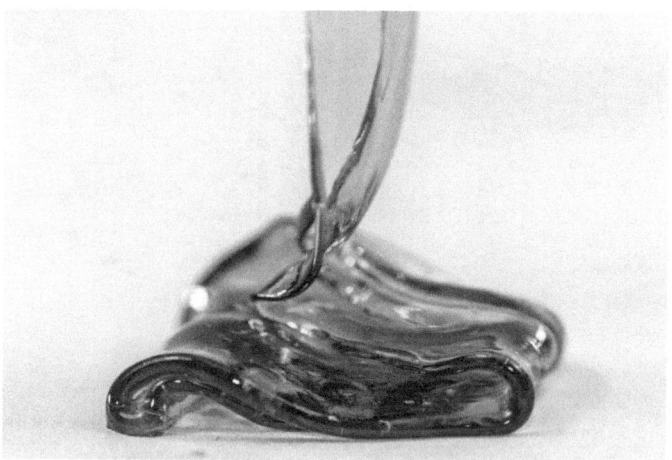

Figure 9.2 Butane hash oil (BHO).

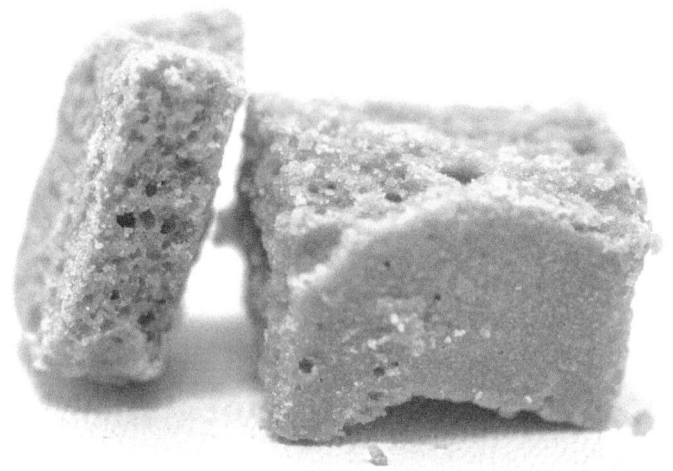

Figure 9.3 Wax.

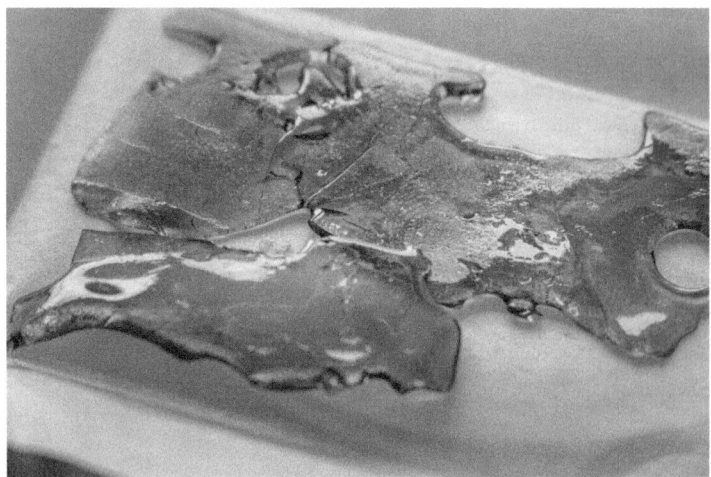

Figure 9.4 Shatter.

Advantages of Cannabis Concentrates

- Increased potency for patients requiring higher cannabinoid doses
- Large doses can be administered quickly
- If inhaled, there is no risk of plant matter entering the lungs

Disadvantages of Cannabis Concentrates

- Increased cost to patient
- Higher risk of overmedicating
- May contain trace amount of solvents
- Processing may remove minor cannabinoids and terpenes
- May contain higher concentration of pesticides

FORMS OF MEDICATION

Smoking

- ***Onset:*** Immediate
- ***Duration:*** 1 to 3 hours
- ***Bioavailability:*** 10% to 25% or 2% to 56%

Smoke absorbs into the bloodstream in seconds. Onset is immediate, and decay is predictable, which makes titration easily achievable. New patients are advised to wait for 15 minutes between inhalations to avoid overconsumption or unwanted psychoactivity.

Fast Facts

Holding cannabis smoke in your lungs does not increase the absorption rate. In fact this only increases the absorption of more harmful compounds.

Cannabis smoke contains over 1,500 chemicals, including some of the same carcinogens found in tobacco, yet there is no conclusive evidence that cannabis smoke contributes to emphysema, cancer, or other adverse effects on pulmonary function. Three decades of research led by Donald Tashkin, MD, director of the pulmonary function laboratories at the University of California, Los Angeles, found that long-term smokers of cannabis had no increased incidence of head, neck, or lung cancers. They also had much lower incidence of these cancers than nonsmokers.

Fast Facts

A recent survey of people who smoked marijuana daily, for up to 20 years, found no evidence that smoking harmed their lungs.

Advantages of Smoking Cannabis

- Rapid onset
- Ease of titration
- Short and predictable duration of effects
- No investment to begin medicating
- Little to no maintenance required

Disadvantages of Smoking Cannabis

- Nonsmokers may find smoke irritating to the lungs
- Burned plant matter produces carbon, tar, and carcinogens
- Inefficient if patient needs higher doses of cannabinoids
- Up to 50% of the active ingredients are incinerated

> **Fast Facts**
>
> *Water pipes (Exhibit 9.1) and bongs deliver larger doses of cannabinoids per inhale than traditional smoking. However, water that cools the smoke can trap therapeutic cannabinoids in the process.*

Vaporization

- ***Onset:*** Immediate
- ***Duration:*** 1 to 3 hours
- ***Bioavailability:*** 10% to 25% or 2% to 56%

Vaporizers heat the oils at a lower temperature than combustion and do not burn plant matter. Since cannabinoids and terpenes heat at temperatures between 340° and 428°F (171° and 220°C), well below the point of combustion, vaporizing is less likely to cause irritating respiratory side effects—it measurably reduces undesirable compounds in smoke.

> **Fast Facts**
>
> *Vaporization is very efficient, as cannabinoids are not incinerated.*

Best practices for vaporizing are simple and straightforward. Inhale, hold for three seconds, and exhale. Note: Because terpenes exhaust before cannabinoids, vaporize after the flavor disappears to get maximum therapeutic effects.

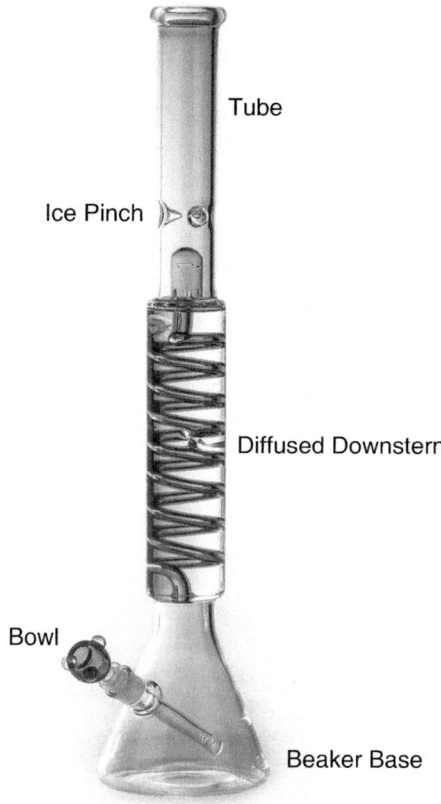

Exhibit 9.1 Anatomy of a water pipe.
Source: © Medical Marijuana 411 (2020).

Types of Vaporizers

- Conduction vaporizer

  - The device heats a metal plate.
  - The metal plate melts the oils similar to a skillet.
  - Some plant matter may be incinerated.

- Convection vaporizer

  - Hot air is circulated around the plant material
  - Oils in the plant material are melted
  - Adjustable temperature
  - Cleaner inhalation with no plant matter

- Oil cartridge vapor pens (Exhibit 9.2)
    - Least expensive option for patients
    - Discreet and easy to use
    - Wide variety of prefilled cartridges for dosing options

> **Fast Facts**
>
> *Vaporizing cannabis flowers allows you to extract the cannabinoids from the dry herb slowly and effectively.*

Advantages of Vaporization

- Vaporized cannabinoids can be inhaled as a cooler, less irritating mist than smoke
- Titration is easy to monitor and adjust
- Allows patient to extract cannabinoids effectively
- No harmful byproducts from smoking
- Higher quality devices are easily cleaned with ethanol

Disadvantages of Vaporization

- Cannabis oils, when vaporized, can clog less sophisticated machines.
- Lower quality devices must be replaced once clogged.
- Vaporizers must be cleaned and maintained.
- Patients will need to learn how to use their machines.

Edibles

- ***Onset:*** 1.5 to 2 hours
- ***Duration:*** 6 to 10 hours
- ***Bioavailability:*** 5% to 20%

Edibles do not provide immediate relief, but they do provide stronger, longer lasting relief than inhaled cannabis—6 to 9 hours depending on the material and a patient's own endocannabinoid system (ECS). The process of passing through the gastrointestinal tract, and being metabolized in the liver before ultimately being absorbed into the bloodstream, changes delta-9-THC into delta-11-THC, an entirely different, longer lasting, and more powerful compound. This difference is significant: Smoking results in only 20% of delta-9-THC metabolizing into delta-11-THC, whereas ingestion results in 100%.

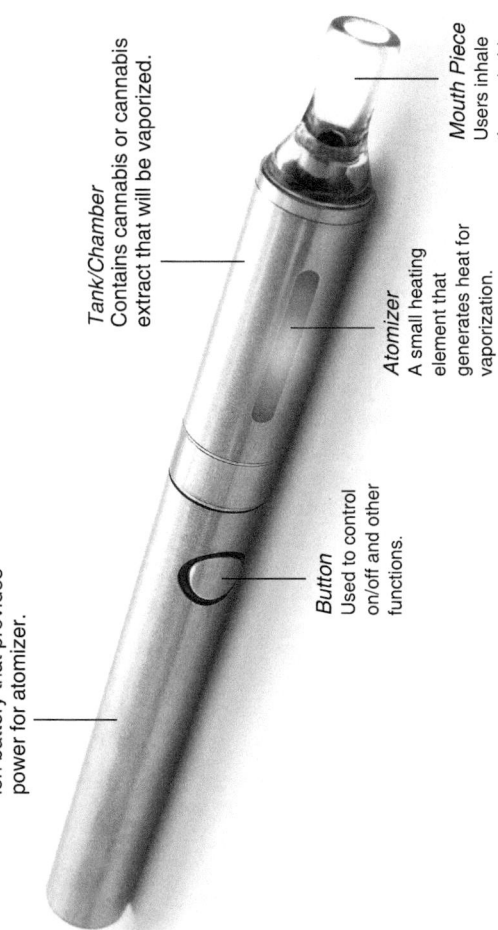

Exhibit 9.2 Anatomy of a vape pen
Source: © Medical Marijuana 411 (2020).

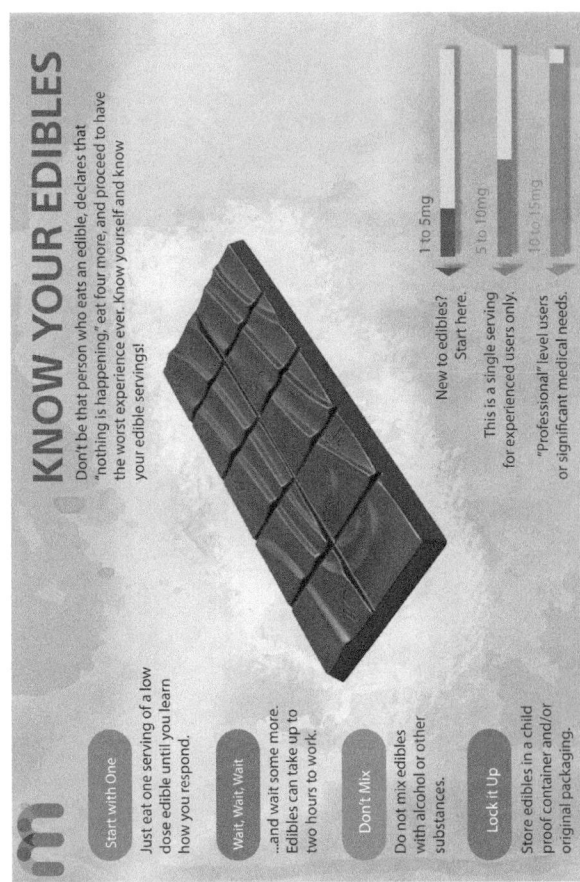

Exhibit 9.3 Edibles Guide
Source: © Medical Marijuana 411 (2020).

Fast Facts

Patients new to edibles must be aware of dose size. Overconsuming edibles can lead to accidental cannabis poisoning.

The primary challenge with edibles is dose titration. Too small a dose produces no relief, and too large a dose can produce extreme psychoactivity, which can result in paranoia and discomfort. Since the onset time is so long, it may take several attempts for a patient to find an optimal dose (Figure 9.5). This is why it is important for patients, especially inexperienced patients, to "start low, go slow."

Fast Facts

Edibles come in a variety of forms: candies, gummy bears, chocolates, cookies, pills, and lozenges.
These types of products create a high risk in environments with children and must be secured properly.

Advantages of Edibles

- Long duration and stronger effects
- Dosing may be easier for a patient to consume
- Eliminates risk associated with smoking
- Exact cannabinoid dosing can be achieved

Disadvantages of Edibles

- Onset of effects is delayed considerably by absorption through the gastrointestinal tract
- Edible products may be made with sugar, which can present complications with diabetic patents.
- Patients may overconsume due to the long onset time.
- Serving size may need to be reduced based on patient's tolerance.
- There is a high risk of accidental cannabis poisoning to children and pets.
- Manufacturing practices may put a patient with food allergies at risk.

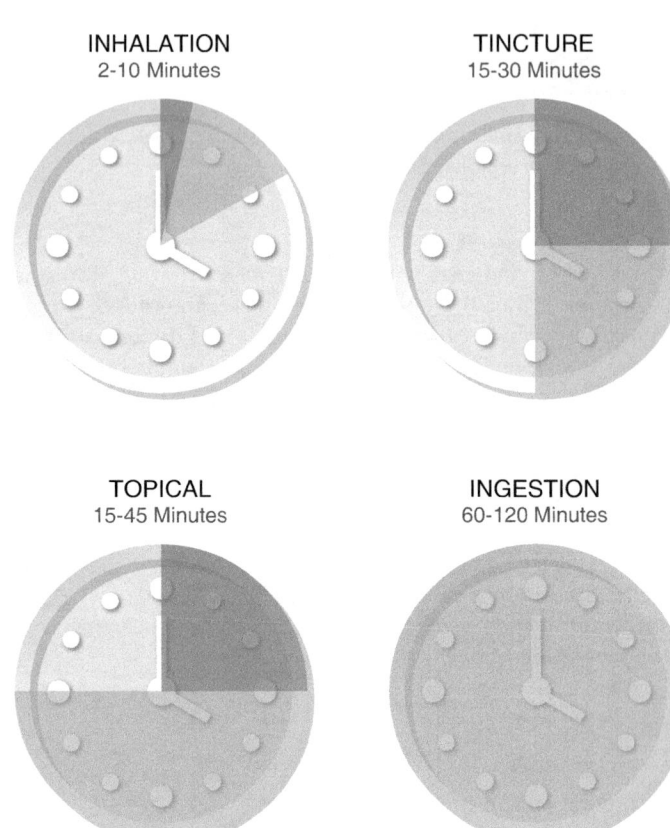

Figure 9.5 Onset time guide.
Source: © Medical Marijuana 411 (2020).

Oral Mucosal: Tinctures, Sprays, Sublingual Drops

- ***Onset:*** 1 to 15 minutes if held in mouth; 1.5 hours if swallowed
- ***Duration:*** 2 to 8 hours
- ***Bioavailability:*** 1% to 12%

Oral mucosal tinctures and extracts are easy to use and reflect the full chemical spectrum of the plant. Even better, they come in various ratios of CBD:THC, which makes dosing for experienced and inexperienced users easy to monitor and adjust.

> **Fast Facts**
>
> *Epidiolex and Sativex are oral mucosal formulations of cannabinoids.*

The best method of taking an oral mucosal tincture, or extract, is to drop or spray some under the tongue, or between the gums and cheek, where a large number of blood vessels reside, and keep it there for a few minutes before swallowing. Avoid drinking or eating anything for 10 minutes following administration. If the tincture is alcohol based, the alcohol could irritate or burn sensitive gums. To lessen irritation, dilute the tincture in water, and swish around the mouth for oral mucosal application. Another option is to dilute the tincture in a liquid oil or medium fat yogurt drink to increase lipophilic absorption.

> **Fast Facts**
>
> *Tinctures held under the tongue will lessen the onset time as the cannabinoids can enter the bloodstream through the blood vessels in the mouth.*

Advantages of Oral Mucosa

- Tinctures are easy to use and titrate
- Various ratios of CBD:THC content are available
- Minor cannabinoids and terpenes are included in some formulations
- Tinctures can be added to food or beverages
- Long shelf-life and flexibility
- Discreet and portable

Disadvantages of Oral Mucosa

- Inconsistencies in labeling on non–FDA-approved formulations
- Delayed onset if swallowed by the patient
- Patients with allergies to carrier ingredients should use caution

Topicals: Creams, Salves, Roll-Ons, Pain Patches

- ***Onset:*** Immediate
- ***Duration:*** 30 minutes to 3 hours
- ***Bioavailability:*** Not applicable

Topicals are available in creams, salves, roll-ons, and patches. Topicals in general do not result in a high typically associated with THC. Topicals are nonpsychoactive unless they contain unusually high amounts of cannabinoids. This is due to CBD crossing the skin barrier more efficiently than THC.

Penetration of the skin barrier can be enhanced by alcohol or lipid media, which is used in longer-duration transdermal patches.

Fast Facts

Topicals are traditionally used to treat targeted areas such as arthritis, inflammation, eczema/psoriasis, acne, and chronic pain.

Advantages of Cannabis Topicals

- Avoids first-pass metabolism by the liver
- Localized pain management
- Reduces inflammation and arthritis
- Nonpsychoactive even when containing THC

Disadvantages of Cannabis Topicals

- Possibility of local irritation
- Low skin penetration of cannabinoids
- Patients with allergies to carrier ingredients should use caution

Suppositories

- ***Onset:*** 15 minutes or less
- ***Duration:*** up to 12 hours
- ***Bioavailability:*** 13% to 67% depending on suppository formulation

Suppositories are extremely efficient but not very popular. They act quickly and efficiently by avoiding first-pass metabolism through the liver, and also provide long-lasting effects. Suppositories are useful for palliative care, treating cancers of pelvic floor, certain GI diseases, menstrual cramps, and for patients who cannot swallow. The depth of insertion is very important: placement past the anal sphincter is key (roughly 1–1.5 inches [2.5–4 cm]).

Fast Facts

Research involving mice who received rectal CBD showed greater relief of colitis symptoms.

Advantages of Cannabis Suppositories

- Avoids first pass of the liver for rapid onset.
- Effects can last up to 12 hours.
- Patients report relief without psychoactivity.
- Ideal for patients who may not be able to ingest or inhale cannabis.
- Can be administered to unresponsive patients.

Disadvantages of Cannabis Suppositories

- Mucosal irritation
- Patient compliance
- GI state may affect absorption

Bibliography

Backes, M. (2014). *Cannabis pharmacy: The practical guide for medical marijuana* (p. 44). New York, NY: Black Dog & Leventhal.

Borgelt, L., Franson, K., Nussbaum, A., & Wang, G. (2013). The pharmacologic and clinical effects of medical cannabis. *Pharmacotherapy, 33*(2), 195–209. doi:10.1002/phar.1187

ElSohly, M. A., Little, T. L. Jr., Hikal, A., Harland, E., Stanford, D. F., & Walker, L. (1991). Rectal bioavailability of delta-9-tetrahydrocannabinol from various esters. *Pharmacology Biochemistry and Behavior, 40*(3), 497–502. doi:10.1016/0091-3057(91)90353-4

ElSohly, M. A., Stanford, D. F., Harland, E. C., Hikal, A. H., Walker, L. A., Little, T. L. Jr., ... Jones, A. B. (1991). Rectal bioavailability of Δ-9-tetrahydrocannabinol from the hemisuccinate ester in monkeys. *Journal of Pharmaceutical Sciences, 80*(10), 942–945. doi:10.1002/jps.2600801008

Fraleigh, N. (2014). *Backdoor medicine: How cannabis suppositories can save lives.* Cannabis Digest. Retrieved from http://cannabisdigest.ca/cannatory/; http://www.alternet.org/drugs/backdoor-medicine-cannabis-suppositories-save-lives

Gieringer, D., St. Laurent, J., & Goodrich, S. (2004). Cannabis vaporizer combines efficient delivery of THC with effective suppression of pyrolytic compounds. *Journal of Cannabis Therapeutics, 4*(1), 7–27. doi:10.1300/J175v04n01_02

Grant, I., Atkinson, J., Gouaux, B., & Wilsey, B. (2012). Medical marijuana: Clearing away the smoke. *The Open Neurology Journal, 6*(1), 18–25. doi:10.2174/1874205X01206010018

Huestis, M. (2007). Human cannabinoid pharmacokinetics. *Chemistry & Biodiversity, 4*(8), 1770–1804. doi:10.1002/cbdv.200790152

Loflin, M., & Earleywine, M. (2014). A new method of cannabis ingestion: The dangers of dabs? *Addictive Behaviors, 39*(10), 1430–1433. doi:10.1016/j.addbeh.2014.05.013

Mannila, J., Järvinen, T., Järvinen, K., Tarvainen, M., & Jarho, P. (2005). Effects of RM-β-CD on sublingual bioavailability of Δ9-tetrahydrocannabinol in rabbits. *European Journal of Pharmaceutical Sciences, 26*(1), 71–77. doi:10.1016/j.ejps.2005.04.020

Mattes, R., Shaw, L., Edling-Owens, J., Engelman, K., & Elsohly, M. A. (1993). Bypassing the first-pass effect for the therapeutic use of cannabinoids. *Pharmacology Biochemistry and Behavior, 44*(3), 745–747. doi:10.1016/0091-3057(93)90194-x

Melamede, R. (2005). Cannabis and tobacco smoke are not equally carcinogenic. *Harm Reduction Journal, 2*, 21. doi:10.1186/1477-7517-2-21

Pletcher, M., Vittinghoff, E., Kalhan, R., Richman, J., Safford, M., Sidney, S., ... Kertesz, S. (2012). Association between marijuana exposure and pulmonary function over 20 years. *JAMA, 307*(2), 173–181. doi:10.1001/jama.2011.1961

Scully, C. (2007). Cannabis; adverse effects from an oromucosal spray. *British Dental Journal, 203*(6), E12. doi:10.1038/bdj.2007.749

Tashkin, D. (2015). Does cannabis pose risks for chronic airflow obstruction? *Annals of the American Thoracic Society, 12*(2), 235–236. doi:10.1513/AnnalsATS.201412-581ED

Wallace, M., Marcotte, T., Umlauf, A., Gouaux, B., & Atkinson, J. H. (2015). Efficacy of inhaled cannabis on painful diabetic neuropathy. *The Journal of Pain, 16*(7), 616–627. doi:10.1016/j.jpain.2015.03.008

Whiteley, N. (2016). *Chronic relief: A guide to cannabis for the terminally and chronically ill*. Austin, TX: Alivio LLC.

10

Side Effects of Cannabis Use

This chapter discusses the adverse side effects of marijuana and marijuana products. It also discusses the risks of developing chronic conditions such as cannabinoid hyperemesis syndrome (CHS) and marijuana use disorder.

In this chapter, you will learn how to:

- Discuss the short- and long-term side effects of cannabis use.
- Explain the contraindications of medicinal cannabis and safety concerns with its use.
- Identify signs of abuse, misuse, and chronic effects of marijuana use.

EFFECTS OF MARIJUANA AND MARIJUANA PRODUCTS

The short- and long-term effects of marijuana consumption can fluctuate from person to person.

Factors That Affect Reaction to Cannabis

- Amount consumed
- Previous cannabis experience
- Age
- Interval between uses

After marijuana is inhaled through the lungs, cannabinoids enter the bloodstream and target the brain and most organs, as well as the nervous system and immune system. However, if consumed orally (by food or beverage), it may take longer for the body to absorb the THC. Thirty to 90 minutes may pass before effects begin. Users may experience heightened sensory perception, or the enhancement of primary senses. Marijuana overactivates parts of the brain that contain the highest number of endocannabinoid receptors. This causes the "high" that people feel.

Fast Facts

Consuming cannabis orally can take 30 to 90 minutes before the effects are felt.

Short-Term Side Effects

As listed on the National Institute on Drug Abuse (NIDA) site, marijuana overactivates parts of the brain that contain the highest number of cannabinoid receptors. Short-term side effects include:

- Altered senses (e.g., seeing brighter colors)
- Altered sense of time
- Changes in mood
- Impaired body movement
- Difficulty with thinking and problem-solving
- Impaired memory
- Hallucinations (when taken in high doses)
- Delusions (when taken in high doses)
- Paranoia and psychosis (when taken in high doses) (NIDA, 2018)

Fast Facts

Consuming more than the recommended dose of an edible product is the leading cause of experiencing paranoia and psychosis.

Long-Term Side Effects

Similar to the lack of clinical studies investigating therapeutic qualities of cannabinoids, only limited studies are available regarding the long-term effects of marijuana. In addition, many of the current studies regarding long-term side effects do not account for the use of cigarettes or other illicit drug use. This can pose a significant public health concern, especially for vulnerable populations such as pregnant women and adolescents. NIDA lists the following wide range of side effects depending on the frequency and duration of use. These effects can be both physical and mental.

PHYSICAL EFFECTS

- Breathing problems
- Increased heart rate
- Problems with child development during and after pregnancy
- Intense nausea and vomiting
- Risk of stroke

Breathing Problems

Marijuana smoke irritates the lungs, and people who smoke marijuana frequently can have the same breathing problems as those who smoke tobacco such as daily cough and phlegm, more frequent lung illness, and a higher risk of lung infections. A study of volunteers suggested that smoking cannabis in a joint form can result in four times the exposure to carbon monoxide and three to five times more tar deposition than smoking a single cigarette. This may be due to the fact that cannabis smokers generally inhale the smoke more deeply than cigarettes and hold the smoke in their lungs longer.

Fast Facts

Unlike heavy tobacco smokers, heavy cannabis smokers exhibit no obstruction of the lung's small airways.

Researchers so far have not found a higher risk for lung cancer in people who smoke marijuana. A 2015 study pooled data on 2,159 lung cancer cases and 2,985 controls from six case–control studies, four of which were unpublished. Among all study participants, there was no statistically significant difference in the risk of lung cancer for habitual cannabis smokers as compared with nonhabitual smokers (odds ratio [OR], 0.96, 95% confidence interval [CI] = 0.66–1.38). Similarly, among participants who did not smoke tobacco, the risk of lung cancer was not significantly higher or lower for habitual cannabis smokers than for nonhabitual cannabis smokers (OR, 1.03, 95% CI = 0.51–2.08).

Fast Facts

While researchers have shown some cannabis smoke–induced cellular damage, they have been unable to demonstrate a link between cannabis smoke and lung cancer.

Increased Heart Rate

Marijuana raises the heart rate for up to 3 hours after smoking, possibly increasing the chance of heart attack. Older people and those with heart problems may be at higher risk. The acute cardiovascular effects of cannabis include increases in heart rate, supine blood pressure, and postural hypotension. Smoking cannabis decreases exercise test duration on maximal exercise tests and increases the heart rate at submaximal levels of exercise.

Fast Facts

Smoking cannabis can raise the resting heart rate, dilate blood vessels, and make the heart pump harder.

Problems With Child Development During and After Pregnancy

There is substantial evidence of a statistical association that marijuana use during pregnancy is linked to lower birth weight. A study of 9,521 mothers showed a 84.20 gram reduction in birth weight for the children of mothers who had used cannabis at least once per week before and throughout pregnancy versus nonusers. However, when adjusted for other drug use such as cocaine or opiates, there was no significant association between cannabis use and lowered birth rate.

> **Fast Facts**
>
> *All studies of cannabis use and pregnancy involved women who were polysubstance drug users.*

There is an increased risk of both brain and behavioral problems in babies. If a pregnant woman uses marijuana, the drug may affect certain developing parts of the fetus' brain. Children exposed to marijuana in the womb have an increased risk of problems with attention, memory, and problem-solving compared with unexposed children.

Cannabinoids are fat-soluble; therefore, they may be present in the fetus and breast milk. Pregnancy, planned pregnancy, or breastfeeding are strong relative contraindications to the use of marijuana.

Intense Nausea and Vomiting

Regular, long-term marijuana use increases the risk of developing cannabinoid hyperemesis syndrome (CHS). This causes users to experience regular cycles of severe nausea, vomiting, and dehydration, sometimes requiring emergency medical attention.

Stroke

Reports have suggested that risk of stroke may increase with cannabis use. The cardiovascular effects of smoking cannabis have been proposed as a possible mechanism. In a 2015 study of 64 patients, 34 cases reported an 81% temporal relationship between cannabis and the indexed event. However, half of the patients also had concomitant stroke risk factors such as tobacco use (34%) and alcohol consumption (11%). Additional reports support the causal link between cannabis and cerebrovascular events. However, concomitant risk factors in each study may account for the cerebrovascular event. At this time there is limited evidence of statistical association between cannabis use and risk of stroke.

> **Fast Facts**
>
> *Between 2010 and 2014, the incidence of stroke steadily increased in recreational marijuana users while it remained flat in the larger population.*

Additional Physical Effects

Due to the increased use of cannabis, healthcare providers should consider other physical effects and stay up-to-date on research as to the risk factors they pose to patients. Cannabis users who orally inhale smoke have higher occurrences of oral health effects such as xerostomia (dry mouth), leukoedema, gingival enlargement, and chronic inflammation of the oral mucosa. Cannabis use may contribute to erectile dysfunction and sexual health concerns in men. Discontinuing heavy cannabis use showed measures of sleep disturbance in cannabis users. At this time, there is limited evidence of statistical association between cannabis use and these physical effects due to the fact that many of the current studies contain concomitant risk factors such as tobacco, alcohol, and illicit drug use.

MENTAL EFFECTS

Long-term marijuana use has been linked to mental illness in some people, such as:

- Temporary hallucinations
- Temporary paranoia
- Worsening symptoms in patients with schizophrenia

Fast Facts

THC has been shown to produce anxiety and psychotic effects, especially in higher doses, whereas CBD has been shown to produce anxiolytic and antipsychotic effects.

Marijuana use has been linked to mental health problems among teens, such as depression, anxiety, and suicidal thoughts. However, study findings have been mixed. Note that national survey studies suggest that it is not uncommon for individuals with mental health disorders to use substances of abuse and, likewise, that it is not uncommon for individuals who abuse or are dependent on drug substances to also meet diagnostic criteria for a mental health disorder. In a 2014 national survey, almost 8 million adults in the United States reported co-occurring substance abuse and mental health disorders.

Persons with a personal or strong family history of psychosis, schizophrenia, or panic disorder have a relative contraindication to using cannabis products containing THC.

WHAT TO AVOID

- Marijuana may cause dizziness, drowsiness, and/or impaired judgment, so users should avoid engaging in potentially hazardous activity. This includes, but is not limited to, driving and operating other heavy machinery.
- Consuming alcohol after marijuana may further enhance any dizziness, drowsiness, or impaired judgment. Users should reduce or avoid alcohol intake after the use of cannabis, especially ingestible products.
- Conversely, cannabis and other cannabis-infused products can enhance dizziness, drowsiness, and/or impaired judgment from other drug substances, including antidepressants, alcohol, antihistamines, sedatives, pain relievers, anxiety medicines, seizure medicines, and muscle relaxants.

Cannabis and Driving

Marijuana, like alcohol, negatively affects a number of skills required for safe driving. Marijuana use can slow down reaction time and the ability to make decisions. High-dose cannabis is associated with decreased mean speed, increased mean and variability in headways, and long reaction times. Several studies have shown increased crash and culpability risks, even after adjusting for such confounders as age, sex, risky behaviors, and polypharmacy. Increased blood THC concentrations and driving within an hour after smoking were strongly associated with higher crash and culpability risks. Human laboratory-controlled drug-administration studies showed THC-induced driving-performance decrements within the first hour that lasted ≥2 hours after smoking, results that are largely consistent with epidemiologic data.

HEALTH EFFECTS OF MARIJUANA ABUSE

Like other substances, marijuana has the potential to be abused. There have been no reported cases of overdose resulting in death due to cannabis use, but healthcare providers should caution about substantial risks such as the risk of poisoning, developing CHS, and/or marijuana use disorder.

Unintentional Cannabis Overdose

With the increased number of states that have legalized medical or recreational marijuana, the availability of cannabis has increased the risk of unintentional cannabis overdose injuries. Children who may consume cannabis edibles, beverages, or candies inadvertently are the most at risk. Colorado Department of Public Health and Environment found moderate evidence that more unintentional pediatric cannabis exposures have occurred in states with increased legal access to cannabis and that the exposures can lead to significant clinical effects requiring medical attention. Several studies report that unintentional pediatric cannabis exposure is associated with potentially serious symptoms, including respiratory depression or failure, tachycardia and other cardiovascular symptoms, and temporary coma.

National Poison Data System found that between 2000 and 2013, U.S. poison centers received 1,969 calls related to cannabis exposure among children younger than 6 years. Most exposures were unintentional (92.2%) and occurred as a result of ingesting cannabis or a cannabis product (75.0%).

Reported Symptoms of Unintentional Cannabis Overdose

- Drowsiness
- Lethargy
- Coma
- Cardiovascular symptoms
- Respiratory depression

Cannabinoid Hyperemesis Syndrome

A new clinical condition known as CHS has emerged, coinciding with the increasing rates of cannabis use, most commonly in individuals with a long history of chronic marijuana use. Symptoms include severe nausea, abdominal pain, and vomiting. Knowledge of the epidemiology, pathophysiology, and natural course of CHS is limited.

As the availability of marijuana increases in legalized states, this condition requires further investigation. Cannabis concentrates and access to products containing higher levels of cannabinoids may lead to an increase in occurrences of CHS in patients.

Fast Facts

Patients suffering from CHS report that they find relief through bathing or showering with hot water.

Marijuana Use Disorder

In 2013, the *Diagnostic and Statistical Manual of Mental Disorders*, Fifth Edition (*DSM-5*; American Psychiatric Association [APA], 2013) defined marijuana use disorder as "occurring when the recurrent use of marijuana causes clinically and functionally significant impairment, such as health problems, disability, and failure to meet major responsibilities at work, school, or home" (APA, 2013).

Symptoms of marijuana use disorder include:

- Disruptions in functioning due to cannabis use
- Development of marijuana tolerance
- Cravings for cannabis
- Development of withdrawal symptoms, such as the inability to sleep, restlessness, nervousness, anger, or depression within a week of ceasing heavy use

In 2015, an estimated 4 million people in the United States met the diagnostic criteria for marijuana use disorder. About 138,000 individuals voluntarily sought treatment. Recent data suggest that 30% of heavy marijuana users may have some degree of marijuana use disorder. Greater frequency of cannabis use increases the likelihood of developing problems. Studies suggest that 9% of users become addicted to marijuana and that number increases to a 17% addiction rate if the user begins in their teens. This is in comparison with 32% of tobacco users, 17% of cocaine users, and 15% of alcohol users.

Illicit Drug Addiction Rates

- Cannabis 9%
- Alcohol 15%
- Cocaine 17%
- Tobacco 32%

Symptoms of Overuse, Abuse, and Addiction

- Regular use of marijuana—daily or several times a day
- Developing an urgency to use marijuana; not being able to focus until after consumption
- Using more and more marijuana to feel the same effects as before
- Consuming larger amounts of marijuana than expected
- Experiencing withdrawal symptoms when not using
- Missing or refraining from usual social and recreational activities
- Interference with work, school, and other responsibilities
- Maintaining a steady supply of marijuana is a priority, especially when exhibiting patterns of hasty behavior to obtain (e.g., lying, stealing, using money you do not have)

References

American Psychiatric Association. (2013). *Diagnostic and statistical manual of mental disorders, fifth edition*. Washington, DC: American Psychiatric Association.

National Institute of Drug Abuse. (2018). *Marijuana*. National Institute on Drug Abuse. Retrieved from https://www.drugabuse.gov/publications/drugfacts/marijuana

Bibliography

Anthony, J. V., Warner, L. A., & Kessler, R. C. (1994). Comparative epidemiology of dependence on tobacco, alcohol, controlled substances and inhalants: Basic findings from the National Comorbidity Survey. *Experimental and Clinical Psychopharmacology, 2*(3), 244–268. doi:10.1037/1064-1297.2.3.244

Benowitz, N. L., & Jones, R. T. (1981). Cardiovascular and metabolic considerations in prolonged cannabinoid administration in man. *The Journal of Clinical Pharmacology, 21*(S1), 214S–223S. doi:10.1002/j.1552-4604.1981.tb02598.x

Bolla, K. I., Lesage, S. R., Gamaldo, C. E., Neubauer, D. N., Funderburk, F. R., Cadet, J. L., … Benbrook, A. R. (2008). Sleep disturbance in heavy marijuana users. *Sleep, 31*(6), 901–908. doi:10.1093/sleep/31.6.901

Cho, C. M., Hirsch, R., & Johnstone, S. (2005). General and oral health implications of cannabis use. *Australian Dental Journal, 50*(2), 70–74. doi:10.1111/j.1834-7819.2005.tb00343.x

Colorado Department of Public Health and Environment. (2015). *Monitoring health concerns related to marijuana use in Colorado: 2014*. Denver, CO: Colorado Department of Public Health and Environment.

Cougle, J. R., Hakes, J. K., Macatee, R. J., Chavarria, J., & Zvolensky, M. J. (2015). Quality of life and risk of psychiatric disorders among regular users of alcohol, nicotine, and cannabis: An analysis of the National Epidemiological Survey on Alcohol and Related Conditions (NESARC). *Journal of Psychiatric Research, 66–67*, 135–141. doi:10.1016/j.jpsychires.2015.05.004

Fergusson, D. M., Horwood, L. J., Northstone, K., & ALSPAC Study Team. Avon Longitudinal Study of Pregnancy and Childhood. (2002). Maternal use of cannabis and pregnancy outcome. *BJOG, 109*(1), 21–27. doi:10.1111/j.1471-0528.2002.01020.x

Galli, J. A., Sawaya, R. A., & Friedenberg, F. K. (2011). Cannabinoid hyperemesis syndrome. *Current Drug Abuse Reviews, 4*(4), 241–249.

Goldschmidt, L., Day, N. L., & Richardson, G. A. (2000). Effects of prenatal marijuana exposure on child behavior problems at age 10. *Neurotoxicology and Teratology, 22*(3), 325–336. doi:10.1016/s0892-0362(00)00066-0

Grotenhermen, F. (2003). Pharmacokinetics and pharmacodynamics of cannabinoids. *Clinical Pharmacokinetics, 42*(4), 327–360. doi:10.2165/00003088-200342040-00003

Hackam, D. (2015). Systematic appraisal of case reports. *Stroke, 46*, 852–856. doi:10.1161/STROKEAHA.115.008680

Hartman, R. L., & Huestis, M. A. (2013). Cannabis effects on driving skills. *Clinical Chemistry, 59*(3), 10. doi:10.1373/clinchem.2012.194381

Hasin, D. S., Saha, T. D., Kerridge, B. T., Goldstein, R. B., Chou, S. P., Zhang, H., ... Grant, B. F. (2015). Prevalence of marijuana use disorders in the United States between 2001–2002 and 2012–2013. *JAMA Psychiatry, 72*(12), 1235–1242. doi:10.1001/jamapsychiatry.2015.1858

Institute of Medicine. (1999). *Marijuana and medicine: Assessing the science base*. Washington, DC: The National Academies Press.

Joshi, S., & Ashley, M. (2016). Cannabis: A joint problem for patients and the dental profession. *British Dental Journal, 220*(11), 597–601. doi:10.1038/sj.bdj.2016.416

Lenne, M. G., Dietze, P. M., Triggs, T. J., Walmsley, S., Murphy, B., & Redman, J. R. (2010). The effects of cannabis and alcohol on simulated arterial driving: Influences of driving experience and task demand. *Accident Analysis & Prevention, 42*(3), 859–866. doi:10.1016/j.aap.2009.04.021

The National Academies of Sciences, Engineering, and Medicine, Health and Medicine. (2017). *The health effects of cannabis and cannabinoids: The current state of evidence and recommendations for research*. Washington, DC: The National Academies Press.

Onders, B., Casavant, M. J., Spiller, H. A., Chounthirath, T., & Smith, G. A. (2016). Marijuana exposure among children younger than six years in the United States. *Clinical Pediatrics, 55*(5), 428–436. doi:10.1177/0009922815589912

Rafaelsen, O. J., Bech, P., & Rafaelsen, L. (1973). Simulated car driving influenced by cannabis and alcohol. *Pharmakopsychiatrie, Neuro-Psychopharmakologie, 6*, 71–83. doi:10.1055/s-0028-1094370

Rajanahally, S., Raheem, O., Rogers, M., Brisbane, W., Ostrowski, K., Lendvay, T., & Walsh, T. (2019). The relationship between cannabis and male infertility, sexual health, and neoplasm: A systematic review. *Andrology, 7*(2), 139–147. doi:10.1111/andr.12585

Renaud, A. M., & Cormier, Y. (1986). Acute effects of marihuana smoking on maximal exercise performance. *Medicine & Science in Sports & Exercise, 18*(6), 685–689. doi:10.1249/00005768-198612000-00014

Richardson, G. A., Ryan, C., Willford, J., Day, N. L., & Goldschmidt, L. (2002). Prenatal alcohol and marijuana exposure: Effects on neuropsychological outcomes at 10 years. *Neurotoxicology and Teratology, 24*(3), 309–320. doi:10.1016/s0892-0362(02)00193-9

Schempf, A. H., & Strobino, D. M. (2008). Illicit drug use and adverse birth outcomes: Is it drugs or context. *Journal of Urban Health, 85*(6), 858–873. doi:10.1007/s11524-008-9315-6

Wang, G. S., Roosevelt, G., & Heard, K. (2013). Pediatric marijuana exposures in a medical marijuana state. *JAMA Pediatrics, 167*(7), 630–633. doi:10.1001/jamapediatrics.2013.140

Wolff, V., Armspach, J. P., Lauer, V., Rouyer, O., Ducros, A., Marescaux, C., & Gény, B. (2015). Ischaemic strokes with reversible vasoconstriction and without thunderclap headache: A variant of the reversible cerebral vasoconstriction syndrome? *Cerebrovascular Diseases, 39*(1), 31–38. doi:10.1159/000369776

Wu, T. C., Tashkin, D. P., Djahed, B., & Rose, J. E. (1988). Pulmonary hazards of smoking marijuana as compared with tobacco. *The New England Journal of Medicine, 318*(6), 347–351. doi:10.1056/NEJM198802113180603

Zhang, L. R., Morgenstern, H., Greenland, S., Chang, S. C., Lazarus, P., Teare, M. D., … Hung, R. J. (2015). Cannabis smoking and lung cancer risk: Pooled analysis in the International Lung Cancer Consortium. *International Journal of Cancer, 136*(4), 894–903. doi:10.1002/ijc.29036

V

Chronic Pain Management

11
Causes of Chronic Pain

Causes of chronic pain are highly variable. There is no clear rationale of why only some patients with acute pain from an injury or condition then go on to develop chronic pain. This chapter discusses the different types of chronic pain a patient may experience.

In this chapter, you will learn how to:

- Describe the types of chronic pain conditions.
- List the different attributes of chronic pain.
- Learn the various pathophysiologic causes of perceived pain.

EPIDEMIOLOGY OF CHRONIC PAIN

The progression from acute to chronic pain is complex and individualized. Patients bridge from acute to chronic pain when pain persists beyond the expected time frame for resolution and recovery from tissue injury. Some conditions, such as lower back pain (LBP), are marked by recurrent "flare-ups" of acute pain with only mild or no intervening symptoms. The most common body areas for chronic pain are lower back, hip, neck, shoulder, and then the knees, in that order.

- In 2016, 20% to 28% of the U.S. population experienced chronic pain.
- About 8% of the population had what is called high-impact chronic pain that affects at least one major life activity.
- The incidence of chronic pain increases as we get older, reaching a peak in the 70s.

Fast Facts

The annual cost of chronic pain in the United States, including healthcare expenses, lost income, and lost productivity, was estimated to be $560 billion in 2016.

CLASSIFICATION OF PAIN

- Acute versus chronic—based on duration of pain
  - Acute pain vanishes once the underlying cause of pain is alleviated and usually does not last longer than 6 months.
  - Chronic pain is pain that is ongoing and usually lasts longer than 6 months.

Nociceptive

Often well localized, nociceptive pain includes somatic, myofascial, or musculoskeletal pain. Nociceptive pain also includes visceral pain from smooth muscles and internal hollow organs. This is usually a referred pain.

Causes of nociceptive pain include:

- Bruises
- Burns
- Fractures
- Pain caused by overuse or joint damage

Neuropathic

Neuropathic pain is caused by a lesion or disease in the somatosensory nervous system. Neuropathic pain typically includes numbness, hypersensitivity, tingling, or paresthesia.

Causes of neuropathic pain include:

- Injuries that can cause lasting nerve damage
- Infection
- Surgery
- Disease

Inflammatory

Inflammatory pain is the result of the localized release of immune mediators at the site of tissue inflammation or injury. It includes soreness, stiffness, and palpable swelling, usually localized to a joint or injured tissue.

Causes of chronic inflammatory pain include:

- Infection
- Untreated injuries
- Autoimmune disorders
- Long-term exposure to irritants
- Smoking
- Obesity
- Alcohol
- Chronic stress

Fast Facts

The immune system plays a critical role in both the development and maintenance of several chronic pain syndromes. The involvement of the immune system includes the release of autoantibodies, or via cytokines, chemokines, and other inflammatory mediators. Additionally, immune cells such as T cells and microglia clearly play key roles in immune-related pain.

RISK FACTORS FOR DEVELOPING CHRONIC PAIN

The risk factors for developing chronic pain are not well established. There is good support for preexisting depression and anxiety increasing the risk of developing chronic pain. This causation probably occurs through neural mechanisms associated with the "stress" associated with the pain. Also, the link between the presence of chronic pain and the onset of depression is well established, probably also through neural mechanisms.

There is also the hypothesis that among persons experiencing "stressful" early life events, altered function of the hypothalamic–pituitary–adrenal axis may be an important mediator of pain onset, and this has been confirmed in a prospective population-based study. Risk is likely to involve both genetic and environmental effects although it is likely that many genes, all with small effects, are involved.

> **Fast Facts**
>
> *A review of 11 studies of nonspecific LBP revealed that 33% of patients "totally" recovered in the first 3 months, but in that group 72% still report episodes of LBP a year later.*

CHRONIC PAIN DIAGNOSIS

Chronic pain persists or recurs for more than 3 months. A subjective, unpleasant, sensory, and emotional experience associated with actual or potential tissue damage and chronic pain may be perceived as a disease in its own right, known as chronic primary pain. In chronic pain syndromes, pain is the sole or main complaint.

Secondary pain syndromes are clearly sequelae to an underlying disease or condition. They include:

- Chronic cancer-related pain
- Chronic neuropathic pain
- Chronic visceral pain
- Chronic posttraumatic and postsurgical pain
- Chronic headache
- Chronic musculoskeletal pain

The *International Classification of Diseases* (ICD-10) did not have a systematic representation of chronic pain conditions, impeding accurate epidemiological investigations and studies of treatment. The new *ICD-11* implements new codes to help improve classification and diagnostic coding for chronic pain conditions that recognize primary pain conditions such as complex regional pain syndrome (CRPS) and fibromyalgia (FM) from those conditions where chronic pain is secondary to an underlying disease or trauma.

PRIMARY PAIN SYNDROMES

Fibromyalgia

A common chronic widespread pain disorder, FM is considered to be the prototypical central chronic pain syndrome. However, use of the term *central* should not suggest that peripheral nociceptive input does not contribute to the sensation of pain; rather, the patient feels more pain than typically would be expected based on the degree of nociceptive input. Unlike nociceptive and neuropathic pain, which are associated with identifiable tissue or nerve damage, the pain of FM is less clear but may result from neurochemical imbalances in the central nervous system (CNS) that lead to an augmentation of pain perception, typified by allodynia (pain due to a stimulus that does not usually provoke pain) and hyperalgesia (increased pain from a stimulus that usually provokes pain). The trigger for FM pain is often difficult or impossible to pinpoint. CNS factors play an important role that involves several mechanisms, including central sensitization or a decrease in descending inhibition.

FM symptoms include:

- Widespread pain in muscles and joints
- Fatigue
- Lack of energy
- Trouble sleeping
- Depression or anxiety
- Memory problems
- Headaches
- Muscle twitches or cramps
- Numbness or tingling
- Itching or burning of the skin

Similar findings of hyperalgesia and allodynia have been observed in other chronic pain states, including irritable bowel syndrome (IBS), overactive bladder, temporomandibular joint (TMJ) syndrome, myofascial pain syndrome, and osteoarthritis (OA)—suggesting that similar CNS changes that play a key role in FM are present in a number of other chronic pain conditions.

Fast Facts

Many cannabinoid investigators now consider FM to be a clinical endocannabinoid deficiency syndrome (CEDS) that results in increased central pain messaging.

Complex Regional Pain Syndrome

CRPS, formerly known as reflex sympathetic dystrophy (RSD), is a chronic pain condition. Type I (originally called RSD) occurs after an illness or injury with no direct evidence of nerve damage in the affected limb. This is approximately 90% of CRPS patients. Type II (causalgia) has distinct evidence of a nerve injury.

CRPS symptoms include:

- Continuous burning or throbbing pain
- Sensitivity to touch or cold
- Swelling of the area
- Skin temperature changes
- Skin color changes
- Skin texture changes
- Hair and nail growth changes
- Joint stiffness, swelling, and damage
- Muscle spasms, tremors, weakness, and loss (atrophy)
- Loss of mobility of the affected area

It is proposed that inflammation and alteration of pain perception in the CNS play important roles. It has been suggested that persistent pain and the perception of nonpainful stimuli as painful may be caused by inflammatory molecules (interleukin-1 [IL-1], interleukin-2 [IL-2], and tumor necrosis factor-alpha [TNF-alpha]) and neuropeptides (substance P) released from peripheral nerves. This release may be caused by inappropriate messaging between sensory and motor fibers at the affected site.

Nonspecific LBP

The most common cause of chronic pain, LBP is the leading cause of lost days from work and early retirement. The diagnosis of LBP is one of exclusion, where other specific causes of LBP such as radiculopathy, tumor, or infection have been excluded.

Fast Facts

The prevalence of chronic LBP is reported to be 23% with 11% to 12% of the adult population being disabled by LBP.

Any innervated structure in the lumbar spine can cause symptoms of lower back and referred pain into the extremity or extremities. The rate of false-positive findings on imaging studies makes finding the anatomic origin of LBP difficult. For example, evidence of herniated disc material is shown on CT scans, MRI, and/or myelography in 20% to 76% of persons with no sciatica. A cross-sectional study of 149 working men aged 20 to 58 years revealed that 32% of asymptomatic subjects had evidence of disc degeneration, disc bulging or protrusion, facet hypertrophy, or nerve root compression and only 47% of their subjects who experienced LBP had an abnormality identified.

Risk factors for developing LBP include:

- Age
- Fitness level
- Pregnancy
- Weight gain
- Genetics
- Occupational risk factors
- Mental health factors

SECONDARY PAIN SYNDROMES

Chronic Cancer-Related Pain

Cancer-related pain can be caused by cancer, treatment for cancer, or a combination of factors. Tumors, surgery, chemotherapy, radiation therapy, and diagnostic procedures may cause chronic pain.

Younger patients are more likely to have cancer pain and pain flares than older patients. Patients with advanced cancer have more severe pain, and many cancer survivors have pain that continues after cancer treatment ends.

Fast Facts

Phantom limb pain is considered to be neuropathic pain. The role of mirror neurons in the brain has been proposed in the generation of phantom pain.

Chronic Postsurgical or Posttraumatic Pain

Acute pain following surgery or trauma is a predictable, physiological response to tissue damage. Patients prepare for some degree of pain or discomfort but expect that it will pass. However, up to one third of patients undergoing common surgical procedures or local trauma report persistent or intermittent pain of varying severity. Larger surgeries and multiple trauma conditions come with even higher rates of chronic pain. Some specific surgeries, such as inguinal herniorrhaphy, and trauma, such as elbow fractures, are associated with chronic neuropathic pain from local nerve injuries and entrapment.

Chronic Neuropathic Pain

Neuropathic pain is caused by a lesion or disease of the somatosensory system, including peripheral fibers and central neurons. It affects 7% to 10% of the general population. Multiple causes of neuropathic pain have been described, and its incidence is likely to increase in the aging population as incidence of diabetes mellitus, HIV, multiple sclerosis (MS), and survival from cancer after chemotherapy increases.

Somatosensory system allows for the perception of:

- Touch
- Pressure
- Pain
- Temperature
- Position
- Movement
- Vibration

Somatosensory nerves are found in the:

- Skin
- Muscles
- Joints
- Fascia

Somatosensory nerves include thermoreceptors, mechanoreceptors, chemoreceptors, proprioceptors, and nociceptors. These sensory neurons send signals to the spinal cord and eventually to the brain for further processing. Lesions or diseases of the somatosensory nervous system can lead to altered and disordered transmission of sensory signals into the spinal cord and the brain.

The most common conditions associated with neuropathic pain include:

- Postherpetic neuralgia
- Trigeminal neuralgia
- Painful radiculopathy
- Diabetic neuropathy
- HIV infection
- Leprosy
- Amputation
- MS
- Peripheral nerve injury pain
- Stroke

Chronic Headache

Daily or near-daily headache is a common problem. Chronic daily headache (CDH) encompasses primary headaches presenting more than 15 days per month and lasting for more than 4 hours per day for the last 3 months. While migraine headaches can be severe and disabling, they are usually not chronic in nature, but infrequent and episodic.

CDH types include:

- Transformed migraine
- Chronic tension-type headache
- New daily persistent headache

Fast Facts

There are a multitude of causes of chronic headaches that include intracranial pathology; cervicocranial conditions; central neuralgias; and head, neck, and face myofascial origins.

Chronic Visceral Pain

Chronic visceral pain is a common clinical problem, yet far less is known about its mechanisms compared with somatic pains. Visceral pain is defined as pain originating from the internal organs. Abdominal pain is among the main reasons for physician visits, with more than 12 million consultations occurring each year in the United States.

Diseases with visceral pain symptoms include:

- Inflammatory bowel disease
- Pancreatitis
- Irritable bowel syndrome (IBS)
- Functional dyspepsia

Fast Facts

Surveys have shown prevalence rates among adults of 25% for intermittent abdominal pain and 20% for chest pain; 24% of women suffer from pelvic pain.

Functional gastrointestinal disorders underlie the most prevalent forms of visceral pain. IBS, one of these functional disorders, is associated with abdominal pain, discomfort, and altered bowel habits. IBS affects an estimated 10% to 15% of the U.S. population with consequent costs estimated to exceed $40 billion. Dysmenorrhea, severe pelvic pain during menstrual cycles, underlies one of the most common gynecological complaints in young women.

Visceral pain results from activation of nociceptors of the thoracic, pelvic, or abdominal hollow organs. Visceral structures are highly sensitive to distension (stretch), ischemia, and inflammation, but relatively insensitive to other stimuli that normally evoke pain such as cutting or burning. Visceral pain is diffuse, difficult to localize and often referred to a distant, usually superficial, structure. It may be accompanied by symptoms such as nausea and vomiting.

Fast Facts

Chronic pain stems from and elicits profound cognitive and emotional consequences, requiring a biopsychosocial approach to understanding and management.

Chronic Musculoskeletal Pain

Twenty percent of the adult population in the United States lives with significant chronic musculoskeletal pain, with a higher prevalence in women, lower income groups, and persons with mental health diagnoses. Generally, chronic muscle pain diagnoses are determined by careful history taking and clinical examinations that reveal tender muscle at palpation, corresponding to the reported painful areas. Chronic musculoskeletal pain most often presents with pain in several locations, often in adjacent or overlapping anatomic locations, such as the neck and shoulders.

Bibliography

Andersson, G. B. (1999). Epidemiological features of LBP. *Lancet, 354*(9178), 581–585. doi:10.1016/S0140-6736(99)01312-4

Balagué, F., Mannion, A. F., Pellise, F., & Cedraschi, C. (2012). Non-specific low back pain. *Lancet, 379*(9814), 482–491. doi:10.1016/S0140-6736(11)60610-7

Borchers, A. T., & Gershwin, M. E. (2014). Complex regional pain syndrome: A comprehensive and critical review. *Autoimmunity Reviews, 13*(3), 242–265. doi:10.1016/j.autrev.2013.10.006

Brennan, F., Carr, D. B., & Cousins, M. (2007). Pain management: A fundamental human right. *Anesthesia & Analgesia, 105*(1), 205–221. doi:10.1213/01.ane.0000268145.52345.55

Bruce, J., & Quinlan, J. (2011). Chronic post surgical pain. *Reviews in Pain, 5*(3), 23–29. doi:10.1177/204946371100500306

Chenot, J., Greitemann, B., Kladny, B., Petzke, F., Pfingsten, M., & Schorr, S. G. (2017). Non-specific low back pain. *Deutsches Ärzteblatt International, 114*(51–52), 883–890. doi:10.3238/arztebl.2017.0883

Cipta, A. M., Pietras, C. J., Weiss, T. E., & Strouse, T. B. (2015). Cancer-related pain management in clinical oncology. *The Journal of Community and Supportive Oncology, 13*(10), 347–355. doi:10.12788/jcso.0173

Clauw, D. J., Arnold, L. M., & McCarberg, B. H. (2011). The science of fibromyalgia. *Mayo Clinic Proceedings, 86*(9), 907–911. doi:10.4065/mcp.2011.0206

Delitto, A., George, S. Z., Van Dillen, L., Whitman, J. M., Sowa, G. A., Shekelle, P., … Godges J. J. (2012). Low back pain: Clinical practice guidelines linked to the international classification of functioning, disability, and health from the orthopaedic section of the American Physical Therapy Association. *Journal of Orthopaedic & Sports Physical Therapy, 42*(4), A1–A57. doi:10.2519/jospt.2012.42.4.A1

Gatchel, R. J., Bevers, K., Licciardone, J. C., Su, J., Du, Y., & Brotto, M. (2018). Transitioning from acute to chronic pain: An examination of different trajectories of low-back pain. *Healthcare (Basel), 6*(2). doi:10.3390/healthcare6020048

Gerdle, B., Ghafouri, B., Emberg, M., & Larsson, B. (2014). Chronic musculoskeletal pain: Review of mechanisms and biochemical biomarkers as assessed by the microdialysis technique. *Journal of Pain Research, 7*, 313–326. doi:10.2147/JPR.S59144

Halker, R. B., Hastriter, E. V., & Dodick, D. W. (2011). Chronic daily headache: An evidence-based and systematic approach to a challenging problem. *Neurology, 76*(7 Suppl. 2), S37–S43. doi:10.1212/WNL.0b013e31820d5f32.

Itz, C. J., Geurts, J. W., van Kleef, M., & Nelemans, P. (2013). Clinical course of non-specific low back pain: A systematic review of prospective cohort studies set in primary care. *European Journal of Pain, 17*(1), 5–15. doi:10.1002/j.1532-2149.2012.00170.x

Macfarlane, G. J. (2016). The epidemiology of chronic pain. *Pain, 157*(10), 2158–2159. doi:10.1097/j.pain.0000000000000676

Macrae, W. A. (2008). Chronic post-surgical pain: 10 years on. *British Journal of Anaesthesia, 101*(1), 77–86. doi:10.1093/bja/aen099

McGreevy, K., Bottros, M. M., & Raja, S. N. (2011). Preventing chronic pain following acute pain: Risk factors, preventive strategies, and their efficacy. *European Journal of Pain Supplements, 5*(2), 365–372. doi:10.1016/j.eujps.2011.08.013

National Center for Complementary and Integrative Health. (2018). *Defining the prevalence of chronic pain in the United States*. Bethesda, MD: National Institutes of Health.

Pascual, J., Colas, R., & Castillo, J. (2001). Epidemiology of chronic daily headache. *Current Pain and Headache Reports, 5*(6), 529–536.

Russo, E. B. (2008). Clinical endocannabinoid deficiency (CECD): Can this concept explain therapeutic benefits of cannabis in migraine, fibromyalgia, irritable bowel syndrome and other treatment-resistant conditions? *Neuro Endocrinology Letters, 29*(2), 192–200.

Savage, R. A., Whitehouse, G. H., & Roberts, N. (1997). The relationship between the magnetic resonance imaging appearance of the lumbar spine and low back pain, age and occupation in males. *European Spine Journal, 6*(2), 106–114. doi:10.1007/bf01358742

Sheng, J., Liu, S., Wang, Y., Cui, R., & Zhang, X. (2017). The link between depression and chronic pain: Neural mechanisms in the brain. *Neural Plasticity, 2017*, 9724371. doi:10.1155/2017/9724371

Sikandar, S., & Dickenson, A. H. (2012). Visceral pain—The ins and outs, the ups and downs. *Current Opinion in Supportive and Palliative Care, 6*(1), 17–26. doi:10.1097/SPC.0b013e32834f6ec9

Subedi, B., & Grossberg, G. T. (2011). Phantom limb pain: Mechanisms and treatment approaches. *Pain Research and Treatment, 2011*, 864605. doi:10.1155/2011/864605

Totsch, S. K., & Sorge, R. E. (2017). Immune system involvement in specific pain conditions. *Molecular Pain, 13*, 1744806917724559. doi:10.1177/1744806917724559

Treede, R. D., Rief, W., Barke, A., Aziz, Q., Bennett, M. I., Benoliel, R., … Wang, S. J. (2019). Chronic pain as a symptom or a disease: The IASP Classification of Chronic Pain for the International Classification of Diseases (ICD-11). *Pain, 160*(1), 19–27. doi:10.1097/j.pain.0000000000001384

Walker-Bone, K., Reading, I., Coggon, D., Cooper, C., & Palmer, K. T. (2004). The anatomical pattern and determinants of pain in the neck and upper limbs: An epidemiologic study. *Pain, 109*(1–2), 45–51. doi:10.1016/j.pain.2004.01.008

12

Treating Chronic Pain With Opioids

Opioids have been regarded for millennia as among the most effective drugs for the treatment of pain. These drugs are also widely feared and are associated with abuse, addiction, and the social consequences of diversion. At the same time, they are essential medications, the most effective drugs for the relief of pain.

In this chapter, you will learn how to:

- List types of noncancer chronic pain that respond to long-term opioid use.
- Understand how to select appropriate chronic pain patients for long-term use of opioids.
- List adverse effects that occur with chronic use of opioids to control pain.

HISTORY OF OPIOID USE

The exponential increase in the use of opioids for chronic pain can be traced back to the early 1990s. Until then opioids were used almost exclusively for acute severe pain, such as postoperative and postinjury pain, and for end-of-life or malignancy-related pain.

Fast Facts

The use of opioids was largely stigmatized, and seen as a dangerous substance, until the 1990s.

The increase in opioid prescriptions was influenced by reassurances given to physicians by certain pharmaceutical companies and medical societies claiming that the risk of addiction to physician-supervised prescription of opioids was very low. During this time, pharmaceutical companies also began to promote the use of opioids in patients with noncancer chronic pain even though there was a lack of evidence regarding the risk and benefits in these patients. By 1999, 86% of patients using opioids were using them for chronic noncancer pain.

- There are over 150 synthetic opioids now known, most discovered between 1875 and 2000, including meperidine, methadone, fentanyl, and oxycodone.
- Oxycodone was released in 1996 with an aggressive marketing campaign promoting the use of opioids for pain relief.

Fast Facts

About 80% of all prescription opioids and 99% of hydrocodone in the world are prescribed in the United States, which has only 4.6% of the world's population.

PAIN: THE FIFTH VITAL SIGN

In 2001, The Joint Commission on Accreditation of Healthcare Organizations (JCAHO) mandated pain be tracked as the "fifth vital sign." The JCAHO recommended that pain be assessed in all patients similarly to blood pressure, temperature, and pulse. This was followed by an increase in use of opioids for pain control.

Fast Facts

Vital Signs

- Body temperature
- Heart rate or pulse
- Respiratory rate
- Blood pressure
- Pain

Consistent scientific evidence does not support extensive use of opioids for all types of chronic pain. Moreover, life-threatening adverse effects and rapid onset of physical addiction often far exceed the benefits of opioids for anything other than very short-term use. In some cases, long-term use of opioids is associated with a worsening of perceived levels of pain, known as opioid-induced hyperalgesia. This is not to be confused with opioid tolerance or opioid withdrawal-associated hyperalgesia.

CURRENT GUIDELINES FOR OPIOIDS IN NONCANCER CHRONIC PAIN

Progressive increases in opioid-related deaths prompted a significant reappraisal of the role of opioids in treating chronic noncancer pain. Opioid prescribing has decreased since 2012, and many providers stopped initiating opioid therapy, but a subgroup of providers continues to write high-risk initial opioid prescriptions.

In 2011, the Institute of Medicine (IOM) convened an ad hoc committee to address the current state of the science with respect to pain research, care, and education, and to explore approaches to advance the field. The committee reviewed and quantified the public health significance of pain, including the adequacy of assessment, diagnosis, treatment, and management of acute and chronic pain in the United States. The report emphasized the importance of looking at the following factors prior to determining the choice of treatment and drug for pain:

- Socioeconomic status
- Age
- Loss of productivity
- Psychiatric conditions

The adverse effects on quality of life from opioids can often be worse than the functional effects of the pain. Secondary psychiatric issues are often adversely affected or aggravated by chronic opioid use and need to be addressed. Further research in a number of public, healthcare, and social arenas was recommended.

Fast Facts

Chronic pain is among the most frequent reasons for seeking medical attention in the United States. Over 100 million adults in the United States are living with chronic pain.

SCIENTIFIC EVIDENCE FOR USING OPIOIDS FOR CHRONIC PAIN

The indications for using opioids in cancer-related and end-of-life care have been well established for decades. Opioid therapy for the treatment of chronic noncancer pain is controversial due to insufficient evidence of long-term efficacy and the risk of serious harm.

A 2018 meta-analysis of 96 randomized trials, including approximately 26,200 patients with chronic noncancer pain in 42 high-quality trials, compared opioids with placebo and found the use of opioids was associated with a small reduction in pain (a reduction of 0.69 cm on a 10-cm scale), slightly improved physical functioning (weighted mean difference: 2.8 points on a 100-point scale), and an increase in the risk of vomiting (relative risk 3.44, 95% confidence interval: 2.89–4.10) compared with placebo. Opioid use was associated with a similar small benefit when compared with nonopioid medications, though the evidence was from low- to moderate-quality studies.

Fast Facts

The most commonly prescribed oral opioid pharmaceuticals contain 325 mg of acetaminophen because of the synergistic effects of the acetaminophen metabolite on CB1 antinociception.

TYPES OF OPIOID MEDICATIONS

Opioids come in immediate-release/short-acting (IR/SA) and extended-release/long-acting (ER/LA) preparations and can be administered through a wide variety of routes. When used for chronic noncancer pain, the most common routes of administration are oral or transdermal.

Immediate-Release/Short-Acting

- Can be used in the management of chronic noncancer pain
- Have a more rapid onset of action
- Have a shorter duration of effect
- Often used for "breakthrough pain" in addition to ER/LA opioids (see Box 12.1 for a list of IR/SA types)

BOX 12.1 TYPES OF IMMEDIATE-RELEASE/SHORT-ACTING OPIOIDS

Codeine	Nucynta IR (tapentadol IR)
Demerol (meperidine)	Opana IR (oxymorphone IR)
Dilaudid IR (hydromorphone IR [instant release])	Oxycodone IR
Levorphanol	Pentazocine-Naloxone
Morphine IR	Ultram (tramadol IR)

Extended-Release/Long-Acting

- These are often reserved for the management of cancer pain, use in palliative care, or conditions associated with persistent pain that is otherwise disabling and associated with significant functional impairment.
- Most pain experts avoid use of ER/LA opioids in opioid-naive patients because of the greatly increased risk of unintentional overdose.
- They are not indicated for "as-needed" analgesia (see Box 12.2 for a list of ER/LA types).

BOX 12.2 TYPES OF EXTENDED-RELEASE/LONG-ACTING OPIOIDS

Belbuca (buprenorphine)	MS Contin (morphine sulfate ER)
Hysingla ER	Embeda (morphine sulfate, naltrexone ER)
Zohydro ER (hydrocodone ER [extended release])	OxyContin
Exalgo (hydromorphone ER)	Xtampza ER (oxycondone ER)
Arymo ER	Opana ER (oxymorphone ER)
Avinza	Nucynta (tapentadol ER)
Kadian	Conzip
MorphaBond	Ultram ER (tramadol ER)

Abuse-Deterrent Opioid Formulation

Abuse-deterrent opioid formulations (ADFs) were developed to decrease opioid abuse, using a variety of technologies. A number of studies have found reductions in abuse, overdose, and diversion of abuse deterrent OxyContinA (oxycodone hydrochloride). There is no evidence that patients cease drug abuse because of the ADF. Rather, there is an associated increase in the use of and overdose with other opioids, most notably heroin. ADFs do not prevent patients from taking higher doses than prescribed via multiple tablets.

Abuse-deterrent drugs are generally more expensive than nonabuse-deterrent opioids and may not be covered by insurance (see Box 12.3 for a list of ADF types).

Box 12.3 Types of Abuse-Deterrent Opioid Formulations

Food and Drug Administration–Approved ADF

OxyContin	Xtampza ER
Embeda	Arymo ER
Hysingla ER	RoxyBond
MorphaBond ER	

Fast Facts

When possible, opioids should be combined with nonopioid pharmacotherapy and nonpharmacologic therapies as appropriate to achieve therapeutic goals with the lowest effective doses of all medications.

Treatment Considerations

Prior to initiating opioids for the treatment of chronic pain (> 3 months duration), consider if potential benefits of opioid therapy outweigh potential harms. Discuss and get consent from the patient of all risks, benefits, and alternatives to opioid therapy. Note if pain is adversely affecting a patient's function and/or quality of life despite appropriate nonopioid pharmacologic and nonpharmacologic therapy.

CENTERS FOR DISEASE CONTROL AND PREVENTION TREATMENT RECOMMENDATIONS

The Centers for Disease Control and Prevention (CDC) published its authoritative Guideline for Prescribing Opioids for Chronic Pain in 2016. Although these guidelines are not binding by state or federal law, they offer guidance for prescribers and are often utilized by policymakers including federal and local regulators, such as medical boards, in determining the standard of care. In addition, many state medical and pharmacy boards are defining specific rules for the prescription of opioids for acute, subacute, and chronic pain.

When to Initiate or Continue Opioids for Chronic Pain

1. Nonpharmacologic therapy and nonopioid pharmacologic therapy are preferred for chronic pain. Consider opioid therapy only if expected benefits for both pain and function are anticipated to outweigh risks. If opioids are used, combine with nonpharmacologic therapy and nonopioid pharmacologic therapy, as appropriate.
2. Before starting opioid therapy for chronic pain, establish treatment goals with all patients, including realistic goals for pain and function, and consider how therapy will be discontinued if benefits do not outweigh risks. Continue opioid therapy only if there is clinically meaningful improvement in pain and function that outweighs risks to safety.
3. Before starting and periodically during opioid therapy, discuss with patients known risks and realistic benefits of opioid therapy and patient and clinician responsibilities for managing therapy.

Opioid Selection, Dosage, Duration, Follow-Up, and Discontinuation

1. When starting opioid therapy for chronic pain, prescribe IR/SA opioids instead of ER/LA opioids.
2. When opioids are started, prescribe the lowest effective dosage. Be cautious prescribing opioids at any dosage, carefully reassess evidence of individual benefits and risks when increasing dosage equal to 50 morphine milligram equivalents (MME)/day, and avoid increasing dosage equal to 90 MME/day, or carefully justify a decision to titrate dosage equal to 90 MME/day.
3. Long-term opioid use often begins with treatment of acute pain. When opioids are used for acute pain, prescribe the lowest effective dose of IR/SA opioids and prescribe no greater quantity than needed for the expected duration of pain severe enough to require opioids. Three days or less will often be sufficient; more than 7 days will rarely be needed.

4. Evaluate benefits and harms with patients within 1 to 4 weeks of starting opioid therapy for chronic pain or of dose escalation and every 3 months or more frequently. If benefits do not outweigh harms of continued opioid therapy, optimize other therapies and work with patients to taper opioids to lower dosages or to taper and discontinue opioids.

Assessing Risk and Addressing Harms of Opioid Use

1. Before starting and periodically during continuation of opioid therapy, evaluate risk factors for opioid-related harms. Incorporate plan strategies to mitigate risk into the management, including offering naloxone when factors that increase risk for opioid overdose, such as history of overdose, history of substance use disorder, higher opioid dosages (equal to 50 MME/day), or concurrent benzodiazepine use, are present.
2. Review the patient's history of controlled substance prescriptions using state prescription drug monitoring program (PDMP) data to determine whether the patient is receiving opioid dosages or dangerous combinations that put him or her at high risk for overdose. Review PDMP data when starting opioid therapy for chronic pain and periodically during opioid therapy for chronic pain, ranging from every prescription to every 3 months.
3. When prescribing opioids for chronic pain, use urine drug testing before starting opioid therapy, and consider urine drug testing at least annually to assess for prescribed medications as well as other controlled prescription and illicit drugs.
4. Avoid prescribing opioid pain medication and benzodiazepines concurrently whenever possible.
5. Offer or arrange evidence-based treatment (usually medication-assisted treatment with buprenorphine or methadone in combination with behavioral therapies) for patients with opioid use disorder (OUD).

ASSESSING RISK AND ADDRESSING HARMS OF OPIOID USE

Specifically assess the risks of intentional and unintentional overdose, OUD, and other serious adverse effects often associated with prolonged use of opioids, such as hypogonadism, depression, and intractable opioid-induced constipation (OIC). Consider treating adverse opioid effects with additional pharmaceuticals.

Part of the assessment of risk includes a history of substance misuse, abuse, or psychiatric disorder. Review prior prescription use through a state PDMP. A baseline urine drug test (UDT) assesses for current or recent opioid/illicit substance use. Patients who test positive for opioids/illicit substances are considered to be very high risk, and are probably not appropriate for opioid therapy.

Several risk assessment tools have been developed to help identify patients who are at risk for misuse or abuse of prescribed opioids. There are few high-quality studies that have assessed the diagnostic accuracy of these instruments for predicting opioid misuse. The pain medication questionnaire (PMQ) and the screener and opioid assessment for patients with pain (SOAPP) had the best evidence; both were developed and validated in five separate studies (four each of acceptable quality). The current opioid misuse measure (COMM) performed best screening for current misuse, developed and validated in three studies of acceptable quality.

Analyze the history and physical exam, along with the risk assessment tools and UDT to stratify the patient into low, medium, or high risk of opioid misuse and abuse.

Low Risk

- No personal or family history of alcohol or substance abuse, without psychiatric disorders, and/or who are low risk based on screening instruments are low risk for opioid misuse.
- May be managed by primary care clinicians with appropriate monitoring

Medium Risk

- Some family history of substance misuse or a personal history of a psychiatric disorder.
- Require more controls incorporated into the prescribing and monitoring approach.
- May benefit from pain management consultation with appropriate specialist support.

High Risk

- Avoid opioid use in patients who are at the highest risk of opioid misuse, if possible.
- A personal history of substance abuse, overdose, or significant underlying psychiatric disorders.
- If opioid therapy is appropriate, monitor carefully and manage in collaboration with an addiction medicine specialist.
- Opioids should not be prescribed for chronic pain for patients with active untreated addiction.

Once a decision has been made to initiate opioid therapy, the patient should complete a standard "Opioid Agreement and Consent" form, although there is little evidence regarding the efficacy of opioid agreements in decreasing opioid misuse. A systematic review of the literature found four poor- to fair-quality observational studies that compared patients who completed treatment agreements with matched or historical controls without treatment agreements. Opioid misuse was decreased modestly (7%–23%) with the use of a treatment agreement, with or without urine drug testing. Guidelines suggest that opioid agreements are helpful to set patient expectations when initiating opioid therapy.

Fast Facts

One mnemonic that is helpful for setting clinical shared goals is "SMART"—Specific, Measurable, Attainable, Relevant, and Time-limited.

SELECTING OPIOIDS, DOSAGE, DURATION, AND FOLLOW-UP

When starting opioid therapy for chronic pain, prescribe IR/SA opioids instead of ER/LA opioids. This will help establish the necessary morphine milligram equivalents (MME/day) dose. (See Appendix C.)

Use caution when prescribing opioids at any dosage. When starting opioids, prescribe the lowest effective dosage. The clinical potency and effectiveness of opioids can vary unpredictably among patients with some achieving excellent relief with one agent, while others require a different drug. It is not possible to predict the optimal dosing regimen for a given patient. For this reason, titrate the dose by slowly increasing it, typically in no more than 25% to 50% increments as a percentage of the total daily dose. Opioids generally have a fairly linear dose–response curve. The risks of overdose increase with higher doses of opioids, and the risks and benefits of opioid therapy need to be reconsidered with any dose escalation.

> **Fast Facts**
>
> *Clinicians should avoid prescribing opioid pain medication and benzodiazepines concurrently whenever possible.*

Offer a rescue dose of naloxone when factors that increase risk for opioid overdose, such as history of overdose, history of substance use disorder, higher opioid dosages (equal to 50 MME/day), or concurrent benzodiazepine use, are present.

SAFELY DISCONTINUING LONG-TERM OPIOID THERAPY

Therapy may be discontinued for ineffectiveness, development of intolerable side effects, opioid-induced hyperalgesia, or development of OUD. Continue to offer patients who are withdrawn from opioid therapy the opportunity to be treated with nonopioid or nonpharmacologic therapies for their chronic pain. Offer or arrange evidence-based treatment (usually medication-assisted treatment [MAT] with buprenorphine or methadone in combination with behavioral therapies) for patients with OUD.

Even short-term exposure to an opioid can cause physical dependence, which manifests as the appearance of withdrawal symptoms on reduction or discontinuation of therapy. Common withdrawal symptoms include:

- Abdominal pain
- Diarrhea
- Nausea and vomiting
- Lacrimation
- Diaphoresis
- Piloerection
- Mild hypertension and tachycardia
- Anxiety and irritability
- Tremor

The degree of physical dependence is related to the dose and duration of therapy and is the near universal outcome of chronic daily use. Physical dependence does not constitute the presence of a substance use disorder or addiction, but it can complicate attempts to reduce the dosage or discontinue opioid therapy.

> **Fast Facts**
>
> *Patients should be gradually tapered off opioids. The optimal weaning strategy has not been clearly established.*

In general, taper of 25% dose reduction per week to minimize withdrawal symptoms. A more rapid taper of 25% to 50% reductions every few days may become clinically necessary. The weaning rate may be rapid for patients taking high opioid doses and slowed when daily doses approach 60 to 80 MME. When opioids are discontinued because of OUD, patients may require opioid detoxification and may require a formal referral program.

Bibliography

Ali, M. M., Henke, R. M., Mutter, R., O'Brien, P. L., Cutler, E., Mazer-Amirshahi, M., & Pines, J. M. (2019). Family member opioid prescriptions and opioid use disorder. *Addictive Behaviors, 95*, 58–63. doi:10.1016/j.addbeh.2019.02.024

Busse, J. W., Wang, L., Kamaleldin, M., Craigie, S., Riva, J. J., Montoya, L., … Guyatt, G. H. (2018). Opioids for chronic noncancer pain: A systematic review and meta-analysis. *JAMA, 320*(23), 2448–2460. doi:10.1001/jama.2018.18472

Butler, S. F., Cassidy, T. A., Chilcoat, H., Black, R. A., Landau, C., Budman, S. H., & Coplan, P. M. (2013). Abuse rates and routes of administration of reformulated extended-release oxycodone: Initial findings from a sentinel surveillance sample of individuals assessed for substance abuse treatment. *The Journal of Pain, 14*(4), 351–358. doi:10.1016/j.jpain.2012.08.008

Cassidy, T. A., DasMahapatra, P., Black, R. A., Wieman, M. S., & Butler, S. F. (2014). Changes in prevalence of prescription opioid abuse after introduction of an abuse-deterrent opioid formulation. *Pain Medicine, 15*(3), 440–451. doi:10.1111/pme.12295

Chou, R., Fanciullo, G. J., Fine, P. G., Adler, J. A., Ballantyne, J. C., Davies, P., … American Pain Society-American Academy of Pain Medicine Opioids Guidelines Panel. (2009). Clinical guidelines for the use of chronic opioid therapy in chronic noncancer pain. *The Journal of Pain, 10*(2), 113–130. doi:10.1016/j.jpain.2008.10.008

Chou, R., Fanciullo, G. J., Fine, P. G., Miaskowski, C., Passik, S. D., & Portenoy, R. K. (2009). Opioids for chronic noncancer pain: Prediction and identification of aberrant drug-related behaviors—A review of the evidence for an American Pain Society and American Academy of Pain Medicine clinical practice guideline. *The Journal of Pain, 10*(2), 131–146. doi:10.1016/j.jpain.2008.10.009

Coplan, P. M., Kale, H., Sandstrom, L., Landau, C., & Chilcoat, H. D. (2013). Changes in oxycodone and heroin exposures in the National Poison Data System after introduction of extended-release oxycodone with abuse-deterrent characteristics. *Pharmacoepidemiology and Drug Safety, 22*(12), 1274–1282. doi:10.1002/pds.3522

Dowell, D., Haegerich, T. M., & Chou, R. (2016). CDC guideline for prescribing opioids for chronic pain—United States, 2016. *MMWR Recommendations and Reports, 65*(1), 1–49. doi:10.15585/mmwr.rr6501e1

Gourlay, D. L., Heit, H. A., & Almahrezi, A. (2005). Universal precautions in pain medicine: A rational approach to the treatment of chronic pain. *Pain Medicine, 6*(2), 107–112. doi:10.1111/j.1526-4637.2005.05031.x

Heit, H. A., & Gourlay, D. L. (2004). Urine drug testing in pain medicine. *Journal of Pain and Symptom Management, 27*(3), 260–267. doi:10.1016/j.jpainsymman.2003.07.008

Institute of Medicine. (2001). *The National Academies Collection: Reports funded by National Institutes of Health, in Relieving Pain in America: A blueprint for transforming prevention, care, education, and research.* Washington, DC: National Academies Press (U.S.) National Academy of Sciences.

Klinger-Gratz, P. P., Ralvenius, W. T., Neumann, E., Kato, A., Nyilas, R., Lele, Z., ... Zeilhofer, H. U. (2018). Acetaminophen relieves inflammatory pain through CB1 cannabinoid receptors in the rostral ventromedial medulla. *The Journal of Neuroscience, 38*(2), 322–334. doi:10.1523/JNEUROSCI.1945-17.2017

Lawrence, R., Mogford, D., & Colvin, L. (2017). Systematic review to determine which validated measurement tools can be used to assess risk of problematic analgesic use in patients with chronic pain. *British Journal of Anaesthesia, 119*(6), 1092–1109. doi:10.1093/bja/aex316

Ling, W., Mooney, L., & Hillhouse, M. (2011). Prescription opioid abuse, pain and addiction: Clinical issues and implications. *Drug and Alcohol Review, 30*(3), 300–305. doi:10.1111/j.1465-3362.2010.00271.x

Manchikanti, L., & Singh, A. (2008). Therapeutic opioids: A ten-year perspective on the complexities and complications of the escalating use, abuse, and nonmedical use of opioids. *Pain Physician, 11*(2 Suppl.), S63–S88.

Morone, N. E., & Weiner, D. K. (2013). Pain as the 5th vital sign: Exposing the vital need for pain education. *Clinical Therapeutics, 35*(11), 1728–1732. doi:10.1016/j.clinthera.2013.10.001

O'Connell, M., Sandgren, M., Frantzen, L., Bower, E., & Erickson, B. (2019). Medical cannabis: Effects on opioid and benzodiazepine requirements for pain control. *Annals of Pharmacotherapy, 53*(11), 1081–1086. doi:10.1177/1060028019854221

Pappagallo, M., & Sokolowska, M. (2012). The implications of tamper-resistant formulations for opioid rotation. *Postgraduate Medical Journal, 124*(5), 101–109. doi:10.3810/pgm.2012.09.2588

Passik, S. D., & Squire, P. (2009). Current risk assessment and management paradigms: Snapshots in the life of the pain specialist. *Pain Medicine, 10* (Suppl. 2), S101–S114. doi:10.1111/j.1526-4637.2009.00670.x

Reed, K., Day, E., Keen, J., & Strang, J. (2015). Pharmacological treatments for drug misuse and dependence. *Expert Opinion on Pharmacotherapy, 16*(3), 325–333. doi:10.1517/14656566.2015.983472

Rosenblum, A., Marsch, L. A., Joseph, H., & Portenoy, R. K. (2008). Opioids and the treatment of chronic pain: Controversies, current status, and future directions. *Experimental and Clinical Psychopharmacology, 16*(5), 405–416. doi:10.1037/a0013628

Severtson, S. G., Bartelson, B. B., Davis, J. M., Muñoz, A., Schneider, M. F., Chilcoat, H., … Dart, R. C. (2013). Reduced abuse, therapeutic errors, and diversion following reformulation of extended-release oxycodone in 2010. *The Journal of Pain, 14*(10), 1122–1130. doi:10.1016/j.jpain.2013.04.011

Starrels, J. L., Becker, W. C., Alford, D. P., Kapoor, A., Williams, A. R., & Turner, B. J. (2010). Systematic review: Treatment agreements and urine drug testing to reduce opioid misuse in patients with chronic pain. *Ann Intern Med, 152*(11), 712–720. doi:10.7326/0003-4819-152-11-201006010-00004

Tompkins, D. A., & Campbell, C. M. (2011). Opioid-Induced hyperalgesia: Clinically relevant or extraneous research phenomenon? *Current Pain and Headache Reports, 15*(2), 129–136. doi:10.1007/s11916-010-0171-1

U.S. Food and Drug Administration. (2016). *FDA requires strong warnings for opioid analgesics, prescription opioid cough products, and benzodiazepine labeling related to serious risks and death from combined use.* Silver Spring, MD: U.S. Food and Drug Administration.

Watkins, E. A., Wollan, P. C., Melton, L. J., & Yawn, B. P. (2008). A population in pain: Report from the Olmsted County health study. *Pain Medicine, 9*(2), 166–174. doi:10.1111/j.1526-4637.2007.00280.x

Zhu, W., Chernew, M. E., Sherry, T. B., & Maestas, N. (2019). Initial opioid prescriptions among U.S. commercially insured patients, 2012–2017. *The New England Journal of Medicine, 380*(11), 1043–1052. doi:10.1056/NEJMsa1807069

13

Treating Chronic Pain With Cannabinoids

Patients report that pain is the most common ailment for which they use cannabinoids. This chapter provides a brief overview of the role of cannabinoids in treating pain and the latest research studies conducted using cannabinoids as a pain treatment.

In this chapter, you will learn how to:

- Review recent clinical studies supporting the use of cannabinoids in different pain conditions.
- List limitations on clinical studies with regard to treating chronic pain with cannabinoids.
- Discuss central and peripheral effects of cannabinoids on pain, spams, and inflammation.

TREATING CHRONIC PAIN WITH CANNABINOID MEDICATIONS

There are varying levels of scientific support for using cannabinoid medication (CM) in many types of chronic pain:

- Centrally mediated pain
- Sympathetically mediated pain
- Peripheral neuropathies
- Cancer-related pain
- Myofascial pain
- Arthritic pain
- Fibromyalgia (FM)

Cannabinoids have an impact on the following pain conditions:

- Nociception and spasticity in the central nervous system (CNS)
- Inflammation-related pain through peripheral actions
- Emotional response to chronic pain

Today, cannabis's Schedule I classification has handicapped the ability to complete high-quality research studies on its medical potential. However, this trend has been changing, and recently studies and randomized controlled trials (RCT) are being conducted to support the use of CMs in treatment of certain chronic pain conditions. The available research documents various benefits from the use of CMs for chronic pain conditions.

Fast Facts

Cannabinoid preparations can be used for acute pain, but in general there is little if any scientific support for this.

In 2017, the National Academies of Sciences, Engineering, and Medicine published a comprehensive review of recent medical literature including 10,000 recent abstracts to determine their relevance. Priority was given to recently published systematic reviews and primary research that studied one of the committee's 11 prioritized health endpoints. The report concluded that there was conclusive or substantial evidence that cannabis or cannabinoids are effective for the treatment of pain in adults.

The Center for Medicinal Cannabis Research (CMCR) at the University of California released a report in 2017 that reviewed the findings of five RCTs on CMs and four preclinical studies. It concluded that the studies "support the likelihood that cannabis may represent a possible adjunctive avenue of treatment for certain difficult-to-treat conditions like neuropathic pain and spasticity" (p. 20).

CMs should be considered as adjuncts to other Food and Drug Administration (FDA)–approved treatments for the various types of pain. The addition of CM can often lead to similar levels of pain relief and functional improvement with decreased use of more toxic pain medications. This harm reduction is especially true for opioids.

> **Fast Facts**
>
> *Acetaminophen has been used to treat pain for 100 years; however, the mechanism of action was only discovered in the past decade. It exerts its effects on pain and body temperature via the endocannabinoid system (ECS) by the acetaminophen metabolite, N-arachidonoylphenolamine.*

Centrally mediated pain includes several forms of nociception, paresthesia, burning, and numbness including multiple sclerosis (MS)-related pain. FM is at least partially a centrally mediated pain condition even though there is no clear specific pathophysiological therapeutic target. CB1 agonism in the CNS decreases the perceived pain centrally. In addition, 5HT1a agonism by CMs decreases the emotional response to and effects of the pain.

CMs reduce the sensation of burning and paresthesia via transient receptor potential cation channel subfamily V member (TRPV1) receptor agonism. This ECS receptor is also known as the "capsaicin" receptor.

Myofascial and inflammatory pain, such as arthritis, originates in the muscles and joints. CB1 agonism can decrease the pain signaling via afferent dorsal root ganglia. Separately, CB2 agonism can decrease pain related to inflammation and swelling at the peripheral site.

STUDIES OF CM EFFECTS ON PAIN

A RCT of vaporized tetrahydrocannabinol (THC) in 39 patients with central and/or peripheral neuropathic pain despite conventional FDA-approved medications revealed:

- The low dose was as effective as the medium dose.
  - Either medium-dose (3.53% THC) or low-dose (1.29% THC) vaporized THC resulted in a similar ($p > 0.7$) number needed to treat to achieve 30% pain reduction versus placebo.
- Vaporized cannabis may present an effective option for patients with treatment-resistant neuropathic pain.

> **Fast Facts**
>
> *There are several high-quality RCTs underway to examine the efficacy of cannabinoids with chronic regional pain syndrome, postherpetic neuralgia, spinal cord injury, and MS.*

Another RCT of 28 subjects smoked cannabis for HIV-associated neuropathic pain. The subjects had been refractory to at least two analgesic classes.

- Subjects smoked cannabis ranging from 1% to 8% THC four times a day for 5 days.
- Primary outcome was pain intensity measured by the Descriptor Differential Scale (DDS) from baseline.
- Pain relief was greater with cannabis than placebo (median difference in DDS pain intensity change, 3.3 points, effect size = 0.60; $p = 0.016$).
- Subjects achieving at least 30% pain relief with cannabis versus placebo were 0.46 (95% confidence interval [I]: 0.28–0.65) and 0.18 (95% CI: 0.03–0.32), respectively.
- Mood and daily functioning improved to a similar extent during both treatment periods. Smoked cannabis was generally well tolerated.

A RCT was performed with THC extract or THC:cannabidiol (CBD) extracts in 177 patients with intractable cancer-related pain despite high doses of opioids. The primary outcome measure was a Numerical Rating Scale (NRS) score.

- Study revealed a statistically significant ($p < 0.05$) reduction in pain improvement, −1.37 versus −0.69 for THC:CBD extract versus placebo.
- Twice as many patients showed 30% or greater reduction in pain, 43% versus 21%, ($p < 0.05$) versus placebo.
- The THC-only extract did not reach significance (23% vs. 21% with placebo).
- This highlights the importance of knowledge of the THC:CBD dose and ratios.

In another RCT, 24 patients with MS and central pain took dronabinol up to 10 mg a day.

- Median spontaneous pain intensity during the last week of treatment was significantly lower with dronabinol compared with placebo (4.0 vs. 5.0); $p = 0.02$.
- Median pain relief score for 50% pain relief was 3.5 (CI: 1.9–24.8).
- Dizziness was more frequent with dronabinol during the first week of treatment.

Fast Facts

More recently, both THC and CBD have been shown to activate various peroxisome proliferator-activated receptors intracellularly.

Nabiximols is made from extracts of two strains of *Cannabis sativa* resulting in an approximate 1:1 ratio of THC to CBD. It is currently in phase 3 trials in the United States. It was approved in Canada in 2005 for central neuropathic pain and intractable spasticity in MS. It is administered via the oromucosal route.

- An RCT in 66 patients with MS and centrally mediated pain was performed using nabiximols oromucosal spray self-titrated.
- CM was superior to placebo in reducing NRS −2.7 (CI: −3.4–2.0) versus −0.8 (−1.5–0.1).
- It also helped with sleep disturbance.

A recent study of 199 patients treated with nabiximols and 198 with placebo self-titrated over 2 weeks showed a nonsignificant ($p = 0.0854$) improvement in average pain (10.7% vs. 4.5%) but statistically superior improvement in two of three quality-of-life instruments at week 3, and all three instruments at week 5. These results were consistent with those of a similar 2017 study where a randomized placebo-controlled, double-blind clinical trial of nabiximols in 30 subjects with painful diabetic neuropathy revealed improvement in pain scores in both groups, but the difference did not reach statistical significance. Depression was felt to be a major confounder of the study findings.

A survey of 457 Canadian FM patients showed that 13% of them were using a variety of cannabinoid medications for self-medicating with "some therapeutic effect." The Canadian Fibromyalgia Treatment Guidelines state that cannabis should be considered for FM patients with sleep disturbance.

> **Fast Facts**
>
> *Some experts think that migraines and FM, along with other nonpain conditions, may represent clinical endocannabinoid deficiency syndromes (CEDS).*

The immune system cells and certain related organs have significant expression of CB2 receptors. This includes the immune system cells in the CNS, microglial cells, and astrocytes. CMs can have significant therapeutic benefit for inflammatory pain and swelling via CB2 agonism.

- CB2 and CB1 receptors are present in large numbers on mast cells affecting the pro-inflammatory function.
- Apoptosis or induction of cell death of local immune cell populations
- Disruption of the release of cytokines produced by T-helper 1 cells and enhanced production of T-helper 2 cells and helpful cytokines
- Stimulation of CB2 receptors resulting in decreased release of histamine, serotonin, and other pro-inflammatory neurotransmitters
- THC stimulation of CB1 receptors has the opposite effects
- CB1 and CB2 receptors are upregulated in the injured tissue
- CB2 receptors are temporarily present in cell lines where they are usually not present after the onset of inflammation

> **Fast Facts**
>
> *The anti-inflammatory effects of CM work via CB2 receptor actions. Many patients can use CBD-only formulations to achieve therapeutic effects on inflammatory pain and swelling.*

SPASM AND SPASTICITY-RELATED PAIN

Spasm and spasticity contribute to the sensation of pain locally or in a diffuse pattern of stiffness. The ECS tonically regulates the synaptic neurotransmission that controls the signs of spasticity and tremors. CMs positively impact spasms and spasticity centrally even though the exact mechanisms of spasm and spasticity are still not well understood.

> **Fast Facts**
>
> *Mice models of MS spasticity and tremor show beneficial effects of CM.*

The first large-scale study of CMs on MS symptoms was published in 2005. About 630 patients with MS and muscle spasticity were treated with THC extract or placebo for 15 weeks.

- Evidence of a treatment effect on patient-reported spasticity and pain ($p = 0.003$)
- Improvement in spasticity reported in 61%, 60%, and 46% of participants on cannabis extract, delta-9-THC, and placebo, respectively.
- Overall, patients felt that these drugs were helpful in treating their diseases.
- There were no major safety concerns.

Subsequently, several RCTs of nabiximols have been completed. Systematic review by the American Academy of Neurology in 2014 concluded that nabiximols and THC are "probably effective" for central pain and spasms.

> **Fast Facts**
>
> *Epidemiological research suggests that the availability of CMs results in decreased usage of prescription opioids, benzodiazepines, and antidepressants in the population.*

EMOTIONAL RESPONSE

As pain becomes chronic, the emotional response to the effects of the pain and psychosocial consequences become significant factors in the perceived level of pain.

> **Fast Facts**
>
> *Apart from its effects on the ECS, CBD exhibits promiscuous pharmacological activity across a wide range of non-ECS receptors, including being an allosteric modulator of µ- and delta-opioids, dopamine D2, GABAa, and glycine and agonizes several 5HT receptors.*

CBD is a very indiscriminate molecule and affects many receptors within and outside of the ECS. It works indirectly on the ECS by:

- Inhibiting fatty acid amide hydrolase (FAAH) and fatty acid binding proteins (FABPs)
- Increasing the amount of naturally occurring endocannabinoids
- Mediating the increase in serotonin and glutamate levels
- Improving both depression and anxiety via 5HT1a receptors

Selecting a CM for chronic pain conditions requires an understanding of the mechanism of action, pharmacodynamics, and pharmacokinetics of both THC and CBD.

- THC mediates most of its therapeutic effects via CB1 agonism, and results in mostly central mechanisms of action of pain perception centers in the brain, and reduction of afferent pain signaling from the periphery.
- CBD does not agonize CB1 or CB2 to any extent but has anti-inflammatory effects by increasing the levels of naturally occurring endocannabinoids, discussed earlier.
- CBD is a TRPV1 agonist and has antihyperalgesic effects via this ECS receptor as well.

Fast Facts

CBD has an affinity for G protein-coupled receptor 55 (GPR55) and various transient receptor potential (TRP) channels and inhibits adenosine uptake.

For most pain conditions, a balanced one-to-one ratio of CBD to THC is recommended, similar to the nabiximols ratio. However, the THC may trigger well-known adverse effects of dizziness, decreased coordination, paranoia, or anxiety. For this reason, a trial of CBD alone may be considered due to its antihyperalgesic and anti-inflammatory effects, with minimal adverse effects.

Chronic pain patients with prominent mood issues, such as secondary anxiety and depression should also be considered for CBD-only formulation, for therapeutic effects via increased serotonin levels at 5HT1a receptors.

Bibliography

Abrams, D. I. (2018). The therapeutic effects of cannabis and cannabinoids: An update from the National Academies of Sciences, Engineering and Medicine report. *European Journal of Internal Medicine, 49*, 7–11. doi:10.1016/j.ejim.2018.01.003

Bolognini, D., Costa, B., Maione, S., Comelli, F., Marini, P., & Di Marzo, V. (2010). The plant cannabinoid delta-9-tetrahydrocannabivarin can decrease signs of inflammation and inflammatory pain in mice, *British Journal of Pharmacology, 160*(3), pp. 677–687.

Bruni, N., Della Pepa, C., Oliaro-Bosso, S., Pessione, E., Gastaldi, D., & Dosio, F. (2018). Cannabinoid delivery systems for pain and inflammation treatment. *Molecules, 23*(10). doi:10.3390/molecules23102478

Costa, B., Giagnoni, G., Franke, C., Trovato, A. E., & Colleoni, M. (2004). Vanilloid TRPV1 receptor mediates the antihyperalgesic effect of the nonpsychoactive cannabinoid, cannabidiol, in a rat model of acute inflammation. *British Journal of Pharmacology, 143*(2), 247–250. doi:10.1038/sj.bjp.0705920

de Mello Schier, A. R., de Oliveira Ribeiro, N. P., Coutinho, D. S., Machado, S., Arias-Carrión, O., Crippa, J. A., ... Silva, A. C. (2014). Antidepressant-like and anxiolytic-like effects of cannabidiol: A chemical compound of *Cannabis sativa*. *CNS & Neurological Disorders Drug Targets, 13*(6), 953–960. doi:10.2174/1871527313666140612114838

Ellis, R. J., Toperoff, W., Vaida, F., van den Brande, G., Gonzales, J., Gouaux, B., ... Atkinson, J. H. (2008). Smoked medicinal cannabis for neuropathic pain in HIV: A randomized, crossover clinical trial. *Neuropsychopharmacology, 34*(3), 672–680. doi:10.1038/npp.2008.120

Fallon, M. T., Albert Lux, E., McQuade, R., Rossetti, S., Sanchez, R., Sun, W., ... Kornyeyeva, E. (2017). Sativex oromucosal spray as adjunctive therapy in advanced cancer patients with chronic pain unalleviated by optimized opioid therapy: Two double-blind, randomized, placebo-controlled phase 3 studies. *British Journal of Pain, 11*(3), 119–133. doi:10.1177/2049463717710042

Grant, I., Atkins, J. H., Mattison, A., & Coates, T. (2017). Report to the Legislature and Governor of the State of California presenting findings pursuant to SB847 which created the CMCR and provided state funding. Center for Medicinal Cannabis Research, University of California, 2010.

Hanlon, K. E., & Vanderah, T. W. (2010). Constitutive activity at the cannabinoid CB1 receptor and behavioral responses. *Methods in Enzymology, 484*, 3–30. doi:10.1016/B978-0-12-381298-8.00001-0

Iskedjian, M., Bereza, B., Gordon, A., Piwko, C., & Einarson, T. R. (2007). Meta-analysis of cannabis based treatments for neuropathic and multiple sclerosis-related pain. *Current Medical Research and Opinion, 23*(1), 17–24.

Johnson, J. R., Burnell-Nugent, M., Lossignol, D., Ganae-Motan, E. D., Potts, R., & Fallon, M. T. (2010). Multicenter, double-blind, randomized, placebo-controlled, parallel-group study of the efficacy, safety, and tolerability of THC:CBD extract and THC extract in patients with intractable cancer-related pain. *Journal of Pain and Symptom Management, 39*(2), 167–179. doi:10.1016/j.jpainsymman.2009.06.008

Kia, S., & Choy, E. (2017). Update on treatment guideline in fibromyalgia syndrome with focus on pharmacology. *Biomedicines, 5*(2), 20. doi:10.3390/biomedicines5020020

Koppel, B. S., Brust, J. C., Fife, T., Bronstein, J., Youssof, S., Gronseth, G., & Gloss, D. (2014). Systematic review: Efficacy and safety of medical marijuana in selected neurologic disorders: Report of the Guideline Development Subcommittee of the American Academy of Neurology. *Neurology, 82*(17), 1556–1563. doi:10.1212/WNL.0000000000000363

Lau, N., Sales, P., Averill, S., Murphy, F., Sato, S. O., & Murphy, S. (2015). A safer alternative: Cannabis substitution as harm reduction. *Drug and Alcohol Review, 34*(6), 654–659. doi:10.1111/dar.12275

Lichtman, A. H., Lux, E. A., McQuade, R., Rossetti, S., Sanchez, R., Sun, W., ... Fallon, M. T. (2018). Results of a double-blind, randomized, placebo-controlled study of nabiximols oromucosal spray as an adjunctive therapy in advanced cancer patients with chronic uncontrolled pain. *Journal of Pain and Symptom Management, 55*(2), 179.e1–188.e1. doi:10.1016/j.jpainsymman.2017.09.001

Lowin, T., & Straub, R. H. (2015). Cannabinoid-based drugs targeting CB1 and TRPV1, the sympathetic nervous system, and arthritis. *Arthritis Research & Therapy, 17*(1), 226. doi:10.1186/s13075-015-0743-x

Mack, A., & Joy, J. (2000). *Marijuana and muscle spasticity*. Washington, DC: National Academies Press (US).

Malfitano, A. M., Proto, M. C., & Bifulco, M. (2008). Cannabinoids in the management of spasticity associated with multiple sclerosis. *Neuropsychiatric Disease and Treatment, 4*(5), 847–853. doi:10.2147/ndt.s3208

Nagarkatti, P., Pandey, R., Rieder, S. A., Hegde, V. L., & Nagarkatti, M. (2009). Cannabinoids as novel anti-inflammatory drugs. *Future Medicinal Chemistry, 1*(7), 1333–1349. doi:10.4155/fmc.09.93

The National Academies of Sciences, Engineering, and Medicine. (2017). *The health effects of cannabis and cannabinoids*. Washington, DC: National Academies Press (US).

Pernía-Andrade, A. J., Kato, A., Witschi, R., Nyilas, R., Katona, I., Freund, T. F., ... Zeilhofer, H. U. (2009). Spinal endocannabinoids and CB1 receptors mediate C-fiber–induced heterosynaptic pain sensitization. *Science, 325*(5941), 760–764. doi:10.1126/science.1171870

Pryce, G., & Baker, D. (2007). Control of spasticity in a multiple sclerosis model is mediated by CB1, not CB2, cannabinoid receptors. *British Journal of Pharmacology, 150*(4), 519–525. doi:10.1038/sj.bjp.0707003

Rieder, S. A., Chauhan, A., Singh, U., Nagarkatti, M., & Nagarkatti, P. (2010). Cannabinoid-induced apoptosis in immune cells as a pathway to immunosuppression. *Immunobiology, 215*(8), 598–605. doi:10.1016/j.imbio.2009.04.001

Segev, A., Korem, N., Mizrachi Zer-Aviv, T., Abush, H., Lange, R., Sauber, G., ... Akirav, I. (2018). Role of endocannabinoids in the hippocampus and amygdala in emotional memory and plasticity. *Neuropsychopharmacology, 43*(10), 2017–2027. doi:10.1038/s41386-018-0135-4

Ste-Marie, P. A., Fitzcharles, M. A., Gamsa, A., Ware, M. A., & Shir, Y. (2012). Association of herbal cannabis use with negative psychosocial parameters in patients with fibromyalgia. *Arthritis Care & Research, 64*(8), 1202–1208. doi:10.1002/acr.21732

Svendsen, K. B., Jensen, T. S., & Bach, F. W. (2004). Does the cannabinoid dronabinol reduce central pain in multiple sclerosis? Randomized double blind placebo controlled crossover trial. *BMJ, 329*(7460), 253. doi:10.1136/bmj.38149.566979.AE

Wade, D. T., Collin, C., Stott, C., & Duncombe, P. (2010). Meta-analysis of the efficacy and safety of Sativex (nabiximols), on spasticity in people with multiple sclerosis. *Multiple Sclerosis, 16*(6), 707–714. doi:10.1177/1352458510367462

Whiting, P. F., Wolff, R. F., Deshpande, S., Di Nisio, M., Duffy, S., Hernandez, A. V., … Kleijnen, J. (2015). Cannabinoids for medical use: A systematic review and meta-analysis. *JAMA, 313*(24), 2456–2473. doi:10.1001/jama.2015.6358

Wilsey, B., Marcotte, T., Deutsch, R., Gouaux, B., Sakai, S., & Donaghe, H. (2013). Low-dose vaporized cannabis significantly improves neuropathic pain. *The Journal of Pain, 14*(2), 136–148. doi:10.1016/j.jpain.2012.10.009

Zajicek, J. P., Sanders, H. P., Wright, D. E., Vickery, P. J., Ingram, W. M., Reilly, S. M., … Thompson, A. J. (2005). Cannabinoids in multiple sclerosis (CAMS) study: Safety and efficacy data for 12 months follow up. *Journal of Neurology, Neurosurgery, and Psychiatry, 76*(12), 1664–1669. doi:10.1136/jnnp.2005.070136

Zlebnik, N. E., & Cheer, J. F. (2016). Beyond the CB1 receptor: Is cannabidiol the answer for disorders of motivation? *Annual Review of Neuroscience, 39*, 1–17. doi:10.1146/annurev-neuro-070815-014038

VI

Cannabinoids and the Opioid Crisis

14

Cannabinoid and Opioid Interactions

This chapter provides a brief discussion of the interaction between opioids and cannabinoids.

In this chapter, you will learn how to:

- List the areas of the brain where opioids and cannabinoids interact.
- List the benefits of cannabinoids when used with opioids.
- Review therapeutic effects of cannabinoid drugs and opioid weaning and relapse prevention.

DEFINITIONS

To understand the interaction between opioids and cannabinoids, there are some key definitions you need to know.

- *Opioidergic agent* is a substance that acts directly throughout the body on opioid neuropeptides, endorphin, enkephalin, dynorphin, or nociception.
- *Opioidergic system* is the multiple mechanisms by which opioids produce their effects by an action involving various opioid receptor molecules in the brain and body.
- *Endocannabinoid system (ECS)* is involved in maintaining homeostasis, neuroprotection, and other regulatory functions (see Chapter 6, Cannabinoids and Terpenes).

- *Addiction* is a primary, chronic disease of brain reward, motivation, memory, and related circuitry. Dysfunction in these circuits leads to characteristic biological, psychological, social, and spiritual manifestations.

The opioid system consists of three receptors:

- Mu
- Delta
- Kappa

These receptors are activated by endogenous opioid peptides:

- Enkephalins
- Endorphins
- Dynorphins
- Nociception

Opioid drugs bind to these receptors and can act as agonists or antagonists. Besides its key role in many aspects of addiction, the opioid system also plays a part in a diverse range of physiological functions, including:

- Nociception
- Mood control
- Eating behavior
- Cognitive processes

The ECS comprises lipid neuromodulators known as endocannabinoids, including anandamide (AEA) and 2-arachidonoylglycerol (2-AG). AEA and 2-AG are synthesized from phospholipid precursors and act locally as retrograde regulators of synaptic transmission throughout the central nervous system (CNS). These lipids are released by postsynaptic neurons and mainly activate presynaptic cannabinoid receptors to transiently or persistently suppress transmitter release from both excitatory and inhibitory synapses.

Fast Facts

Studies have shown that opioids and cannabinoids work synergistically.

The ECS has enzymes for the synthesis and degradation of the endocannabinoids and two well-characterized receptors, cannabinoid receptors CB1 and CB2. The ECS plays a key role in the modulation of pain response, with processing of central and peripheral pain signals, learning and memory, reward and emotions in response to pain.

Animal models suggest that the CB1 receptors in several centers of the brain are responsible for:

- Modulation of pain perception
- Emotional response to pain
- Reward associated with addiction

The opioidergic system and ECS are parallel systems in many ways and have been shown to interact.

- CB1 receptors and MOR are distributed in many of the same areas of the brain, including the areas for pain:
  - Periaqueductal gray area
  - Ventral tegmental area (VTA)
  - Locus coeruleus
  - Nucleus accumbens
  - Central amygdala
  - Prefrontal cortex
  - Dorsal hippocampus
  - Medial basal hypothalamus

- The regions of the brain that have to do with nociception have high levels of CB1 and mu-opioid receptors (MORs).

MU-OPIOID RECEPTORS

MORs are G-protein-coupled receptors such as CB1 and CB2 receptors. They are the site of action of innate opioids and of opioid medications. Opioid medications reduce pain by binding to and stimulating MOR in the CNS, leading to a decreased perception of pain via inhibition of ascending pain pathways that start in the spinal cord.

Fast Facts

MOR are potent agonists and therefore can cause respiratory depression, the most common cause of opioid overdose death. (See also Figure 14.1.)

MOR are heavily expressed on respiratory neurons in the brainstem. There are essentially no cannabinoid receptors in the brainstem.

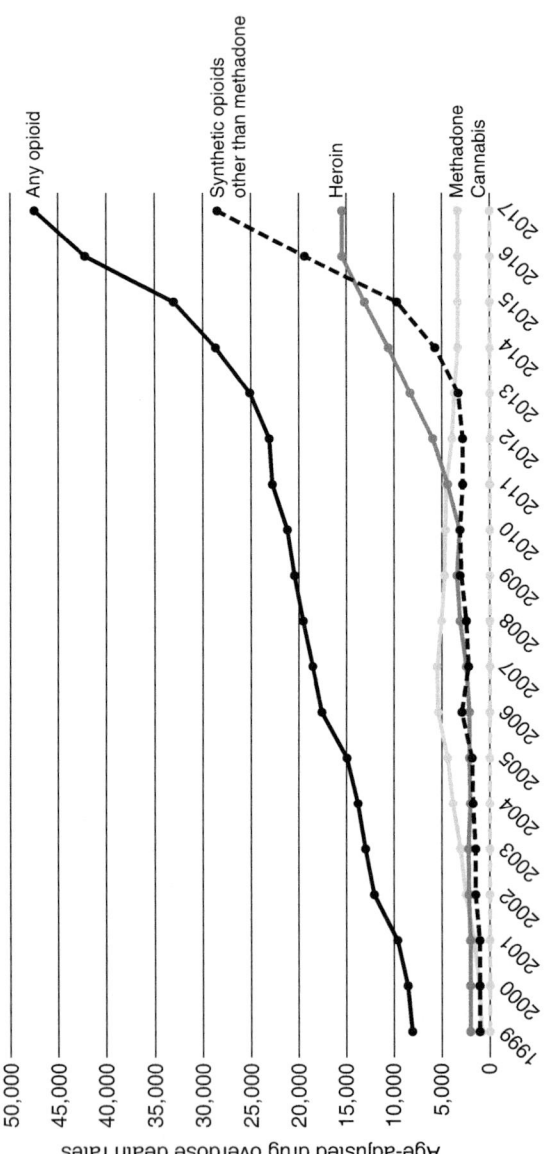

Figure 14.1 Opioid overdose death rates, 1999–2017.
Source: Data from Centers for Disease Control and Prevention WONDER. Retrieved from https://wonder.cdc.gov/mcd.html.

> **Fast Facts**
>
> *Cannabinoids do not act at the respiratory neurons in the brainstem. Cannabinoids do not cause respiratory depression. Cannabinoid use or misuse has not been associated with death from physiologic mechanisms.*

MOR AND INTERACTION WITH CANNABINOID RECEPTORS

Both tetrahydrocannabinol (THC) and cannabidiol (CBD) are allosteric modulators of MOR and delta opioid receptors (DOR) that indirectly amplify the effects of opioids at the mu-opioids binding site. This effect is associated with observed synergistic effects of cannabis and opioid medications.

Stimulation of CB1 receptors significantly affect the rewarding properties of opioids, and vice versa. Both MOR and CB1 receptors are reciprocally involved with the developments of condition place preference (CPP), an animal model for drug use reward. This overlapping involvement in reward is partially mediated by cannabinoid and opioid disinhibition of the dopamine systems of the VTA.

> **Fast Facts**
>
> *Both the opioidergic system and the ECS play a major role in the control of pain as well as in mood regulation, reward processing, and the development of addiction.*

In addition to support for the role of the ECS in the rewarding effects of opioids, this overlapping effect results in the lessening of opioid tolerance. In animal models, CB1 agonists help alleviate several symptoms of opioid withdrawal, including escape jumps, diarrhea, paw tremors, and weight loss. CB1 receptors agonism also improves of the affective symptoms of dysphoria and negative affect, which is mediated via kapa opioid receptors (KOR).

THC, when used with morphine, has been shown to impact the two most important hallmarks of opioid use disorder (OUD)—dose escalation and physical dependence—by reducing the development of tolerance and desensitization of the MOR receptors.

> **Fast Facts**
>
> *Cannabinoids appear to lessen opioid tolerance and negative effects of dysphoria.*

Conflicting data on the involvement of CB1 in opioid reward and withdrawal mean further preclinical and clinical research is necessary to evaluate mechanistic insights into the involvement of the ECS and the opioidergic system. It could be that CBD and THC impact opioid reward and withdrawal via allosteric mechanisms on MOR and KOR.

USING CANNABINOID MEDICATION AND OPIOIDS TOGETHER

Cannabinoid medication (CM) and opioid medications can be used in combination.

- Adjunct medication to decrease or spare the amount of the opioid medications used for pain control
- Decrease the reward associated with opioid addiction and relapse.
- Decrease the unpleasant adverse effects associated with opioid withdrawal.
- Alleviate the anxiety and depression associated with chronic opioid use.

Animal models have shown that modulation of CB1 receptors have a profound effect on the rewarding properties of opioids and vice versa. The mutual involvement in reward and addiction is modulated at least partially by opioid and/or cannabinoid disinhibition of the dopamine neurons in the VTA. This is a well-characterized mechanism in the rewarding properties of drugs of abuse and other addictive behaviors.

> **Fast Facts**
>
> *There are specific opioid–cannabinoid interactions in the modulation of neurochemical effects as well as behavioral responses associated with reward and relapse.*

There is abundant animal model research for the importance of CB1 receptors in the rewarding effects of opioids and amelioration of tolerance. Yet numerous preclinical studies have shown that CB1 agonists readily alleviate the transient symptoms of opioid withdrawal in animal models, conflicting with the previously discussed rewarding properties of CB1 agonism and opioids. Mechanistic effects outside of the ECS have been postulated. Unfortunately, there are no well-designed clinical trials of clearly defined cannabinoid ratios and doses of CMs in opioid withdrawal. However, an observational study of 116 heroin and cocaine users evaluated the reduction of opioid-withdrawal symptoms during 10 weeks of methadone dose tapering. The investigators did not find statistically different self-reporting of opioid-withdrawal symptoms among the 46 cannabis users.

Fast Facts

Genetic polymorphisms can play a role in as much as 30% to 50% of the risk of drug addiction through many mechanisms.

CMs and opioids can be used separately or together for analgesia, in addition to a wide variety of other classes of analgesic oral and topical drugs. Indeed, 90% of patients in state-regulated medical cannabis registries list chronic pain as the qualifying condition (QC). This percentage may be skewed by the fact that chronic pain, along with anxiety, is the second most common QC. Both conditions are highly subjective in nature and easy to feign to obtain a state medical cannabis card. An unreported but significant proportion of these chronic pain patients were already using opioids for chronic pain.

Fast Facts

About 90% of patients in state-regulated medical cannabis registries list chronic pain as the qualifying condition.

Several surveys of patients with chronic pain of all types show that a significant proportion of patients prefer CMs to opioids and decrease the use of opioids by 40% to 60% after adding CMs. Survey respondents noted fewer cognitive adverse effects and better quality of life with CMs.

One retrospective study of motor vehicle accident patients who were already cannabis users suggested that they needed higher doses of opioids for analgesia in acute pain. Chronic cannabis users had significantly higher use of opioids postinjury.

Fast Facts

Preclinical studies have shown that coadministration of opioids and CM attenuates the development of opioid tolerance.

The august National Academies of Sciences, Engineering, and Medicine (2017) also confirmed the efficacy of CMs for chronic pain. Several epidemiologic and observational studies have shown statistically significant reversals in opioid-related deaths linked with medical cannabis laws. Subsequently, many state medical cannabis authorities have added OUD to the list of qualifying conditions to allow patients to obtain medical cannabis, hoping to reduce harm from opioids. However, the available preclinical research suggests that coadministration of CMs and opioids may have synergistic rewarding effects. Further clinical research is necessary on this issue.

Both opioids and CMs risk building tolerance with chronic use. In addition, a subset of chronic users of both drug types develops physical dependence and withdrawal symptoms during abstinence. The cannabis-withdrawal symptoms are similar to those produced with nicotine withdrawal.

OPIOID SPARING

CMs and opioids can be coadministered to reduce the amount of the more detrimental opioid drug being used for analgesia. Human studies have shown that subanalgesic doses of THC and morphine, when coadministered, significantly reduce pain. Other studies confirmed a truly synergistic mechanism behind opioid sparing and enhanced analgesia with CM.

In addition, several studies have shown that adjunct CM decreases opioid consumption or prevents opioid dose escalation. The mechanisms underlying CM alternation of opioid consumption are yet to be determined. Although these findings are promising, several other studies have shown that CM use either has no impact on opioid consumption or may increase nonmedical opioid use.

OPIOID WEANING

Opioid weaning refers to gradually decreasing the dose of opioids without going physiologically into a withdrawal state.

- CMs can be used to increase the analgesic effects of the gradually lowered doses of opioids.
- CMs provide the beneficial effects of analgesia through CB1 receptor mechanisms.
- CMs provide allosteric modulation of opioids on the MOR.
- CMs, and especially CBD, would be expected to help with any mood changes and perceived stress associated with weaning.

OPIOID WITHDRAWAL

Opioid withdrawal refers to the physiological changes associated with abstinence from opioids after chronic use. It results in negative emotional states such as anxiety or irritability when the drug is not accessible, and uncontrolled craving for the drug that interferes with daily activities, despite the emergence of adverse consequences.

Fast Facts

CBD has been shown to reduce the rewarding aspects of multiple drugs of abuse, including opioids and appears to have low reinforcing properties with limited abuse potential and to inhibit drug-seeking behavior.

OPIOID RELAPSE

The most prominent and pervasive problem with OUD treatment is the prevention of relapse. Once weaned off opioids drugs, there is still the underlying addiction, which is considered to be a neuropsychiatric disease. The weaned patients often still maintain compulsive drug-seeking behavior. The relapse rates can reach as high as 85% after 12 months, depending on the type of program or use of medication-assisted treatment (MAT).

- MAT with opioid antagonists and ultra-long acting opioids has been shown to be the most effective in available research.
- MAT with the use of CMs has not been adequately studied.
- Clinical studies of CBD in alcohol or cigarette consumption have yielded mixed results.

> **Fast Facts**
>
> *Animal studies of CBD and cocaine and also alcohol addiction have been promising, showing long-term efficacy after a short course of treatment.*

CBD is a particularly promising CM because of its various therapeutic effects related to relapse, including perceived stress, anxiety, depression, and compulsive activity. CBD has specific beneficial effects on the neurocircuitry of addiction, from "craving," to "binge/intoxication" and finally to "withdrawal" and negative mood. CBD also reduces heroin craving.

> **Fast Facts**
>
> *Genetic studies have revealed significant associations between polymorphisms in both MOR1 and CB1 receptors and association with drug addiction.*

Bibliography

Abrams, D. I., Couey, P., Shade, S. B., Kelly, M. E., & Benowitz, N. L. (2011). Cannabinoid-opioid interaction in chronic pain. *Clinical Pharmacology & Therapeutics, 90*(6), 844–851. doi:10.1038/clpt.2011.188

Allsop, D. J., Copeland, J., Norberg, M. M., Fu, S., Molnar, A., Lewis, J., & Budney, A. J. (2012). Quantifying the clinical significance of cannabis withdrawal. *PLoS One, 7*(9), e44864. doi:10.1371/journal.pone.0044864

Bachhuber, M. A., Saloner, B., Cunningham, C. O., & Barry, C. L. (2017). Medical cannabis laws and opioid analgesic overdose mortality in the United States, 1999–2010. *JAMA Internal Medicine, 174*(10), 1668–1673. doi:10.1001/jamainternmed.2014.4005

Befort, K. (2015). Interactions of the opioid and cannabinoid systems in reward: Insights from knockout studies. *Frontiers in Pharmacology, 6*, 6. doi:10.3389/fphar.2015.00006

Bellnier, T., Brown, G. W., & Ortega, T. R. (2018). Preliminary evaluation of the efficacy, safety, and costs associated with the treatment of chronic pain with medical cannabis. *Mental Health Clinician, 8*(3), 110–115. doi:10.9740/mhc.2018.05.110

Boehnke, K. F., Litinas, E., & Clauw, D. J. (2016). Medical cannabis use is associated with decreased opiate medication use in a retrospective cross-sectional survey of patients with chronic pain. *The Journal of Pain, 17*(6), 739–744. doi:10.1016/j.jpain.2016.03.002

Bolognini, D., Costa, B., Maione, S., Comelli, F., Marini, P., & Di Marzo, V. (2010). The plant cannabinoid delta-9-tetrahydrocannabivarin can decrease signs of inflammation and inflammatory pain in mice, *British Journal of Pharmacology, 160*(3), pp. 677–687.

Degenhardt, L., Lintzeris, N., Campbell, G., Bruno, R., Cohen, M., Farrell, M., & Hall, W. D. (2015). Experience of adjunctive cannabis use for chronic non-cancer pain: Findings from the Pain and Opioids IN Treatment (POINT) study. *Drug and Alcohol Dependence, 147,* 144–150. doi:10.1016/j.drugalcdep.2014.11.031

Epstein, D. H., & Preston, K. L. (2015). No evidence for reduction of opioid-withdrawal symptoms by cannabis smoking during a methadone dose taper. *The American Journal on Addictions, 24*(4), 323–328. doi:10.1111/ajad.12183

Gonzalez-Cuevas, G., Martin-Fardon, R., Kerr, T. M., Stouffer, D. G., Parsons, L. H., Hammell, D. C., ... Weiss, F. (2018). Unique treatment potential of cannabidiol for the prevention of relapse to drug use: Preclinical proof of principle. *Neuropsychopharmacology, 43*(10), 2036–2045. doi:10.1038/s41386-018-0050-8

Gruber, S. A., Sagar, K. A., Dahlgren, M. K., Gonenc, A., Smith, R. T., Lambros, A. M., ... Lukas, S. E. (2019). Frontiers | The grass might be greener: Medical marijuana patients exhibit altered brain activity and improved executive function after 3 months of treatment. *Frontiers in Pharmacology, 8,* 983. doi:10.3389/fphar.2017.00983

Hurd, Y. L., Yoon, M., Manini, A. F., Hernandez, S., Olmedo, R., Ostman, M., & Jutras-Aswad, D. (2015). Early phase in the development of cannabidiol as a treatment for addiction: Opioid relapse takes initial center stage. *Neurotherapeutics, 12*(4), 807–815. doi:10.1007/s13311-015-0373-7

Kathmann, M., Flau, K., Redmer, A., Tränkle, C., & Schlicker, E. (2006). Cannabidiol is an allosteric modulator at mu- and delta-opioid receptors. *Naunyn-Schmiedeberg's Archives of Pharmacology, 372*(5), 354–361. doi:10.1007/s00210-006-0033-x

Koob, G. F., & Volkow, N. D. (2010). Neurocircuitry of addiction. *Neuropsychopharmacology, 35*(1), 217–238. doi:10.1038/npp.2009.110

Livingston, M. D., Barnett, T. E., Delcher, C., & Wagenaar, A. C. (2017). Recreational cannabis legalization and opioid-related deaths in Colorado, 2000–2015. *American Journal of Public Health, 107*(11), 1827–1829. doi:10.2105/AJPH.2017.304059

Lopez-Moreno, J. A., Lopez-Jimenez, A., Gorriti, M. A., & de Fonseca, F. R. (2010). Functional interactions between endogenous cannabinoid and opioid systems: Focus on alcohol, genetics and drug-addicted behaviors. *Current Drug Targets, 11*(4), 406–428. doi:10.2174/138945010790980312

Maldonado, R., Berrendero, F., Ozaita, A., & Robledo, P. (2011). Neurochemical basis of cannabis addiction. *Neuroscience, 181,* 1–17. doi:10.1016/j.neuroscience.2011.02.035

The National Academies of Sciences, Engineering, and Medicine. (2017). *The health effects of cannabis and cannabinoids.* Washington, DC: National Academies Press (US).

Ohno-Shosaku, T., & Kano, M. (2014). Endocannabinoid-mediated retrograde modulation of synaptic transmission. *Current Opinion in Neurobiology, 29*, 1–8. doi:10.1016/j.conb.2014.03.017

Reiman, A., Welty, M., & Solomon, P. (2017). Cannabis as a substitute for opioid-based pain medication: Patient self-report. *Cannabis and Cannabinoid Research, 2*(1), 160–166. doi:10.1089/can.2017.0012

Roberts, J. D., Gennings, C., & Shih, M. (2006). Synergistic affective analgesic interaction between delta-9-tetrahydrocannabinol and morphine. *European Journal of Pharmacology, 530*(1–2), 54–58. doi:10.1016/j.ejphar.2005.11.036

Salottolo, K., Peck, L., Tanner, A., Carrick, M. M., Madayag, R., McGuire, E., & Bar-Or, D. (2018). The grass is not always greener: A multi-institutional pilot study of marijuana use and acute pain management following traumatic injury. *Patient Safety in Surgery, 12*(1), 16. doi:10.1186/s13037-018-0163-3

Shover, C. L., Davis, C. S., Gordon, S. C., & Humphreys, K. (2019). Association between medical cannabis laws and opioid overdose mortality has reversed over time. *Proceedings of the National Academy of Sciences of the United States of America, 116*(26), 12624–12626. doi:10.1073/pnas.1903434116

Singh, M. E., Verty, A. N., McGregor, I. S., & Mallet, P. E. (2004). A cannabinoid receptor antagonist attenuates conditioned place preference but not behavioral sensitization to morphine. *Brain Research, 1026*(2), 244–253. doi:10.1016/j.brainres.2004.08.027

Smith, G. L. (2016). *Medical cannabis: Basic science and clinical applications* (p. 225). Beverly Farms, MA: Aylesbury Press.

Wiese, B., & Wilson-Poe, A. R. (2018). Emerging evidence for cannabis' role in opioid use disorder. *Cannabis and Cannabinoid Research, 3*(1), 179–189. doi:10.1089/can.2018.0022

Wills, K. L., & Parker, L. A. (2016). Effect of pharmacological modulation of the endocannabinoid system on opiate withdrawal: A review of the preclinical animal literature. *Frontiers in Pharmacology, 7*, 187. doi:10.3389/fphar.2016.00187

Wilson, A. R., Maher, L., & Morgan, M. M. (2008). Repeated cannabinoid injections into the rat periaqueductal gray enhances subsequent morphine antinociception. *Neuropharmacology, 55*(7), 1219–1225. doi:10.1016/j.neuropharm.2008.07.038

Zanettini, C., Panlilio, L. V., Aliczki, M., Goldberg, S. R., Haller, J., & Yasar, S. (2011). Effects of endocannabinoid system modulation on cognitive and emotional behavior. *Frontiers in Behavioral Neuroscience, 5*, 57. doi:10.3389/fnbeh.2011.00057

15

Cannabis as an Adjunct to Opioids

There is a growing body of scientific evidence to support the use of cannabinoids as adjuncts to opioids in the treatment of chronic pain, and, to a lesser extent, acute pain. This chapter discusses the use of cannabinoids for opioid sparing.

In this chapter, you will learn how to:

- Understand the various effects that cannabinoids can have that are adjunctive to opioid drugs.
- List adverse effects from long-term use of opioids that may be improved with use of adjunctive cannabinoids.
- Understand how cannabinoids can have adjunctive effects using the endocannabinoid system (ECS), mu-opioid receptors (MORs), and through other non-ECS receptor activity.

CANNABIS AS AN ADJUNCT TO OPIOIDS

When used in conjunction with opioids, cannabinoids can lead to synergistic effects for the relief of pain, resulting in a reduction in the need for opioids. Although it is an emerging area of research, some evidence supports the cannabis–opioid-sparing hypothesis. The safety profile of cannabinoids when used in known doses and titrated by educated patients is far superior to opioids. Concomitant use of cannabinoids can prevent the development of tolerance to and withdrawal from opioids, suggesting increased use of cannabinoids as adjuncts to opioids may lead to harm reduction from prescription opioids. There is limited survey-based contrary evidence to the efficacy of cannabinoids for pain control and opioid reduction, which supports the need for further high-quality trials.

Medical cannabis and Food and Drug Administration (FDA)-approved cannabinoid drugs have various therapeutic effects and may be good adjuncts to ongoing use of opioids drugs.

- Provide pain relief via various mechanisms in the CNS.
- Reduce painful inflammation and spasm at the site of the pain using the ECS.
- Synergistic effects with opioids via allosteric modulation at MORs.
- Improve some of the adverse effects of long-term use of opioids and emotional response to pain via non-ECS receptor effects.
- Cannabinoids can decrease pain perception, decrease inflammation at the site of pain, decrease the emotional response to the pain, and improve the efficiency of opioids at MORs.
- Cannabinoids should be considered as adjunctive to ongoing use of opioids. Several studies suggest that patients gradually reduce opioid use spontaneously with the addition of cannabinoids.
- Cannabinoids can improve symptoms of depression and anxiety through 5HT1a agonism by both tetrahydrocannabinol (THC) and cannabidiol (CBD).
- Adjunctive use of opioids and cannabinoids can result in a reduced rate of opioid tolerance due to desensitized MOR receptors.
- Studies suggest that combined use of opioids and cannabinoids can reduce some of the adverse effects associated with chronic opioid use.

Fast Facts

Cells in injured tissue temporarily express CB2 receptors, when they usually do not express these receptors. These receptors help mediate the inflammatory effects of the injured tissue and reestablish homeostasis.

RECENT STUDIES OF ADJUNCT OPIOID AND CANNABINOID USE

There has been concern that combining opioids and cannabinoids may increase the adverse cognitive effects associated with THC and opioids. However, recent research presented at the 2019 American Society for Pharmacology and Experimental Therapeutics meeting revealed combining cannabinoids with morphine did not significantly increase impulsivity or memory impairment in a Rhesus monkey model. The data provided additional evidence that opioid–cannabinoid mixtures are effective for treating pain and do not have greater, and in some cases have less, adverse effects compared with larger doses of each drug alone.

Dampening of Afferent Spinal Cord Pain Messaging

- In a mouse model, CBD significantly decreased afferent firing and raised pain thresholds.
- It was suggested that CBD desensitized the joint afferent fibers responsible for mechanosensitive nociception.

Decreased Emotional Response to Pain

- Cannabinoid drugs and preparations can decrease the emotional response to chronic pain via 5HT1a stimulation, especially with CBD.
- Cannabinoids, through effects of serotonin and glutamate levels, can also have a positive impact on mood and anxiety, commonly associated with chronic pain.

Allosteric Modulation of MOR

- MOR and CB1 receptors are located in centers related to pain perception, and CB1 stimulation results in allosteric modulation of the MOR that improves the nociceptive effects of natural and pharmacologic opioids at MOR.

Decrease Inflammation Locally at Site of Pain

- CB2 upregulation and improved binding dampens the inflammatory cascade and the cellular inflammatory response.
- This results in less swelling, inflammation, and associated pain from the pain-generating site.

Decrease Spasm and Spasticity Associated With Pain

- Spasms are thought to originate in areas of the brain that control movement, including several sites with abundant cannabinoid receptors.
- Nabiximols, a cannabis extract combination of approximately 1:1 CBD to THC, has been shown in several randomized controlled clinical trials (RCTs) to be effective for control of painful spasm or spasticity in multiple sclerosis (MS) patients.

CONTRARY EVIDENCE

Not all the research supports of the use of cannabinoids as an adjunct. A 4-year prospective study of 1,514 participants who completed baseline interviews and follow-up questionnaires showed that cannabis use was common, and by 4-year follow-up, 295 (24%) of participants had used cannabis for pain.

- Participants who used cannabis had
  - Greater pain severity scores,
  - Greater pain interference scores,
  - Lower pain self-efficacy scores, and
  - Greater generalized anxiety disorder severity scores.
- The study found no evidence that cannabis use reduced prescribed opioid use or increased rates of opioid discontinuation.
- The higher pain levels and lower self-efficacy in managing pain may be significant unaddressed confounders of the study results.

Fast Facts

People who used cannabis had greater pain and lower self-efficacy in managing pain, and there was no evidence that cannabis use reduced pain severity or interference or exerted an opioid-sparing effect.

Another study suggests that many chronic pain patients were "essentially substituting medical cannabis for opioids and other medications for chronic pain treatment and finding the benefit and side effect profile of cannabis to be greater than these other classes of medications" (Boehnke, Litinas, & Clauw, 2016).

One study of 244 medical cannabis patients found:

- Medical cannabis use was associated with a 64% decrease in opioid use
- Decreased number and side effects of medications
- Improved quality of life (45%)

A survey of 2,897 medical cannabis patients using opioids for at least 6 months for chronic pain found that respondents "overwhelmingly reported that cannabis provided relief on *par* with their other medications" (Reiman, Welty, & Solomon, 2017). The other medications and measures of pain relief were not documented.

- About 97% of the respondents "strongly agreed/agreed" that they can decrease the number of opiates they consume when they also use cannabis.
- About 81% "strongly agreed/agreed" that taking cannabis by itself was more effective for treating their condition than taking cannabis with opioids.
- Results were similar for those using cannabis with nonopioid-based pain medications.

Fast Facts

Substances called Cannflavins A, B, and C have been identified in hemp sprouts. Cannflavins A and B have been shown to be potent inhibitors of prostaglandin E2 production in vitro. Cannflavins are currently being studied for their potential use as anti-inflammatory agents.

OTHER ADJUNCTIVE DRUGS

Many classes of drugs, oral and topical, can provide pain relief or improve adverse effects from opioids. NSAIDs, antidepressants, anticonvulsants, and topical analgesic/counter-irritant preparations used in conjunction with opioids reduce the amount of opioid necessary for adequate pain control.

Fast Facts

Palmitoylethanolamide (PEA) is a cannabinoid-like drug that mediates biological activities including activation of cannabinoid receptors. It has been found in several clinical studies to be effective for neuropathic and other types of pain.

SELECTING THE RIGHT CANNABINOID

There are several FDA-approved cannabinoid drugs that fall into two classes. Dronabinol formulations (capsules, or liquid) are pure THC analogues (discussed in Chapter 8, Isolate Cannabinoid Pharmaceuticals). These have their therapeutic effects primarily by acting on CB1 receptors in the ECS. Dronabinol can be effective for pain reduction, but can have adverse effects on cognition and coordination similar to opioids.

The other FDA-approved drug is CBD in an oral preparation (discussed in Chapter 9, Medical Marijuana and Bioavailability). CBD has therapeutic effects by increasing the endocannabinoid tone and dampening the immune inflammatory response. CBD also exerts antinociceptive effects as a transient receptor potential cation channel subfamily V member 1 (TRPV1) antagonist.

Nabiximols is an investigational new drug in the United States, but has been approved as a pharmaceutical drug for MS neuropathic pain and spasticity in other countries for a decade. It is an approximately 1:1 ratio of CBD to THC cannabinoid extract and has had promising phase 3 results for pain and spasticity. Some RCTs have not shown statistically significant improvement in chronic uncontrolled cancer pain.

Fast Facts

Some patients find a balanced ratio helpful for neuropathic pain, rheumatism, and overall mood enhancement.

Medical cannabis preparations come in various ratios that can help with titration and balancing adverse and therapeutic effects. In states with medical marijuana laws, forms of dosing may include inhalation, tinctures, topicals, and edibles that can be acquired with a clinician's recommendation. Preparations with a 1:1 CBD:THC ratio have been found to have the greatest effect on neuropathic pain. Ratios with a greater CBD content, such as a 20:1 ratio, are recommended for pain from inflammation.

Bibliography

Bellnier, T., Brown, G. W., & Ortega, T. R. (2018). Preliminary evaluation of the efficacy, safety, and costs associated with the treatment of chronic pain with medical cannabis. *Mental Health Clinician, 8*(3), 110–115. doi:10.9740/mhc.2018.05.110

Boehnke, K. F., Litinas, E., & Clauw, D. J. (2016). Medical cannabis use is associated with decreased opiate medication use in a retrospective cross-sectional survey of patients with chronic pain. *The Journal of Pain, 17*(6), 739–744. doi:10.1016/j.jpain.2016.03.002

Borgelt, L. M., Franson, K. L., Nussbaum, A. M., & Wang, G. S. (2013). The pharmacologic and clinical effects of medical cannabis. *Pharmacotherapy, 33*(2), 195–209. doi:10.1002/phar.1187

Braida, D., Limonta, V., Malabarba, L., Zani, A., & Sala, M. (2007). 5-HT1A receptors are involved in the anxiolytic effect of Delta 9-tetrahydrocannabinol and AM 404, the anandamide transport inhibitor, in Sprague-Dawley rats. *European Journal of Pharmacology, 555*(2–3), 156–163. doi:10.1016/j.ejphar.2006.10.038

Campbell, G., Hall, W. D., Peacock, A., Lintzeris, N., Bruno, R., Larance, B., … Degenhardt, L. (2018). Effect of cannabis use in people with chronic non-cancer pain prescribed opioids: Findings from a 4-year prospective cohort study. *The Lancet Public Health, 3*(7), 341–350. doi:10.1016/S2468-2667(18)30110-5

Gabrielsson, L., Mattsson, S., & Fowler, C. J. (2016). Palmitoylethanolamide for the treatment of pain: Pharmacokinetics, safety and efficacy. *British Journal of Clinical Pharmacology, 82*(4), 932–942. doi:10.1111/bcp.13020

Grenald, S., Guan, Y., & Raja, S. (2018). Peripheral cannabinoid and mu opioid receptor synergistic inhibition of neuropathic pain. *The Journal of Pain, 19*(3), S74. doi:10.1016/j.jpain.2017.12.169

Kathmann, M., Flau, K., Redmer, A., Tränkle, C., & Schlicker, E. (2006). Cannabidiol is an allosteric modulator at mu- and delta-opioid receptors. *Naunyn-Schmiedeberg's Archives of Pharmacology, 372*(5), 354–361. doi:10.1007/s00210-006-0033-x

Khan, S. P., Pickens, T. A., & Berlau, D. J. (2019). Perspectives on cannabis as a substitute for opioid analgesics. *Pain Management, 9*(2), 191–203. doi:10.2217/pmt-2018-0051

Lopez-Moreno, J. A., Lopez-Jimenez, A., Gorriti, M. A., & de Fonseca, F. R. (2010). Functional interactions between endogenous cannabinoid and opioid systems: Focus on alcohol, genetics and drug-addicted behaviors. *Current Drug Targets, 11*(4), 406–428. doi:10.2174/138945010790980312

Lucas, P. (2012). Cannabis as an adjunct to or substitute for opiates in the treatment of chronic pain. *Journal of Psychoactive Drugs, 44*(2), 125–133. doi:10.1080/02791072.2012.684624

Lucas, P., Baron, E. P., & Jikomes, N. (2019). Medical cannabis patterns of use and substitution for opioids & other pharmaceutical drugs, alcohol, tobacco, and illicit substances; results from a cross-sectional survey of authorized patients. *Harm Reduction Journal, 16*(1), 9. doi:10.1186/s12954-019-0278-6

Mannucci, C., Navarra, M., Pieratti, A., Russo, G. A., Caputi, A. P., & Calapai, G. (2011). Interactions between endocannabinoid and serotonergic systems in mood disorders caused by nicotine withdrawal. *Nicotine & Tobacco Research, 13*(4), 239–247. doi:10.1093/ntr/ntq242

Miller, L. K., & Devi, L. A. (2011). The highs and lows of cannabinoid receptor expression in disease: Mechanisms and their therapeutic implications. *Pharmacological Reviews, 63*(3), 461–470. doi:10.1124/pr.110.003491

Murataeva, N., Miller, S., Dhopeshwarkar, A., Leishman, E., Daily, L., Taylor, X., ... Straiker, A. (2019). Cannabinoid CB2R receptors are upregulated with corneal injury and regulate the course of corneal wound healing. *Experimental Eye Research, 182*, 74–84. doi:10.1016/j.exer.2019.03.011

Nagarkatti, P., Pandrey, R., Rieder, S. A., Hegde, V. L., & Nagarkatti, M. (2009). Cannabinoids as novel anti-inflammatory drugs. *Future Medicinal Chemistry, 1*(7), 1333–1349. doi:10.4155/fmc.09.93

Pacher, P., & Mechoulam, R. (2011). Is lipid signaling through cannabinoid 2 receptors part of a protective system? *Progress in Lipid Research, 50*(2), 193–211. doi:10.1016/j.plipres.2011.01.001

Patel, S., & Hillard, C. J. (2009). Role of endocannabinoid signaling in anxiety and depression. *Current Topics in Behavioral Neurosciences, 1*, 347–371. doi:10.1007/978-3-540-88955-7_14

Philpott, H. T., O'Brien, M., & McDougall, J. J. (2017). Attenuation of early phase inflammation by cannabidiol prevents pain and nerve damage in rat osteoarthritis. *Pain, 158*(12), 2442–2451. doi:10.1097/j.pain.0000000000001052

Pollastro, F., Taglialatela-Scafati, O., Allara, M., Muñoz, E., Di Marzo, V., De Petrocellis, L., & Appendino, G. (2011). Bioactive prenylogous cannabinoid from fiber hemp (Cannabis sativa). *Journal of Natural Products, 74*(9), 2019–2022. doi:10.1021/np200500p

Pu, S., Eck, P., Jenkins, D. J., Lamarche, B., Kris-Etherton, P. M., West, S. G., ... Jones, P. J. (2016). Interactions between dietary oil treatments and genetic variants modulate fatty acid ethanolamides in plasma and body weight composition. *British Journal of Nutrition, 115*(6), 1012–1023. doi:10.1017/S0007114515005425

Reiman, A., Welty, M., & Solomon, P. (2017). Cannabis as a substitute for opioid-based pain medication: Patient self-report. *Cannabis and Cannabinoid Research, 2*(1), 160–166. doi:10.1089/can.2017.0012

Remesic, M., Hruby, V. J., Porreca, F., & Lee, Y. S. (2017). Recent advances in the realm of allosteric modulators for opioid receptors for future therapeutics. *ACS Chemical Neuroscience, 8*(6), 1147–1158. doi:10.1021/acschemneuro.7b00090

Smith, P. A., Selley, D. E., Sim-Selley, L. J., & Welch, S. P. (2007). Low dose combination of morphine and delta 9-tetrahydrocannabinol circumvents antinociceptive tolerance and apparent desensitization of receptors. *European Journal of Pharmacology, 571*(2–3), 129–137. doi:10.1016/j.ejphar.2007.06.001

Vigil, J. M., Stith, S. S., Adams, I. M., & Reeve, A. P. (2018). Associations between medical cannabis and prescription opioid use in chronic pain patients: A preliminary cohort study. *PLoS One, 12*(11), e0187795. doi:10.1371/journal.pone.0187795

Wade, D. T., Collin, C., Stott, C., & Duncombe, P. (2010). Meta-analysis of the efficacy and safety of Sativex (nabiximols), on spasticity in people with multiple sclerosis. *Multiple Sclerosis, 16*(6), 707–714. doi:10.1177/1352458510367462

Wiese, B., & Wilson-Poe, A. R. (2018). Emerging evidence for cannabis' role in opioid use disorder. *Cannabis and Cannabinoid Research, 3*(1), 179–189. doi:10.1089/can.2018.0022

16

Opioid Sparing With Cannabinoids

When used chronically, opioids have considerable side effects, including constipation, impaired sleep, depression, respiratory depression, and risk of unintentional overdose. This chapter reviews the various options for opioid sparing, including the use of cannabinoids, to minimize the side effects of opioid use.

In this chapter, you will learn how to:

- Understand the options of opioid sparing to minimize side effects of chronic use.
- List the categories of drugs used for opioid sparing.
- List the benefits to patients when implementing opioid sparing.

OPIOID SPARING

Decreasing the dose of opioids, via opioid sparing, leads to several harm reduction goals, including fewer accidental overdoses and fewer adverse effects, such as intractable constipation, depression, and hypogonadism. Reducing the Morphine Equivalent Dose (MED) of opioids often decreases the need for other drugs used to treat opioid adverse effects (Table 16.1). At the same time, opioid sparing with other medications should provide similar antinociception.

Table 16.1

Morphine Equivalent Dose	
Opioid (Doses in mg/day Except Where Noted)	Conversion Factor
Codeine	0.15
Fentanyl transdermal (in mcg/hr)	2.4
Hydrocodone	1
Hydromorphone	4
Methadone	
1–20 mg/day	4
21–40 mg/day	8
41–60 mg/day	10
>61–80 mg/day	12
Morphine	1
Oxycodone	1.5
Oxymorphone	3

Note: These dose conversions are estimated and cannot account for all individual differences in genetics and pharmacokinetics.

A wide variety of nonopioid medications are often used to reduce the opioid dose. This is especially true as the MED increases over time. Opioid sparing, while providing similar if not superior pain relief, has several benefits.

- Reduces the cognitive impairment from higher opioid doses
- Reduces adverse effects associated with chronic use of opioids
- Reduces the risk of unintentional overdose that can occur with higher MEDs
- Decreases the rate of opioid tolerance

ACUTE VERSUS CHRONIC OPIOID SPARING

More recently, opioid sparing is being used for acute pain to prevent patients from requiring more than very short-term use of any opioid drugs for moderate to severe postoperative or postinjury pain.

Goal of Opioid Sparing for Acute Pain

- Minimize the opioid-related adverse effects.
- Minimize the possibility of physical dependence on opioids.
- Regional blocks and other interventional pain management procedures are being used to prevent the need for opioids.
- Reduce the number of opioid prescriptions provided at hospital discharge or postoperative discharge.
- Reduce the number of unused opioids diverted to illicit use.
- Reduce the number of patients given several weeks of prescription opioids while awaiting first postdischarge doctor's examination.

Fast Fact

A 2019 study revealed that postoperatively "many patients reported unused opioids, infrequent use of analgesic alternatives, and lack of knowledge regarding safe opioid storage and disposal" (Bicket et al., 2019).

Goal of Opioid Sparing for Chronic Pain

- Provide antinociceptive effects that can result in lower opioid doses.
- Reduce the frequency of opioid doses.
- Slow development of opioid tolerance and physical dependency.

There is little scientific support, or research, to support the efficacy of opioids for chronic pain, especially for neuropathic pain. A 2015 systematic review and meta-analysis of opioids for neuropathic pain reveals that most of the randomized placebo-controlled studies evaluating efficacy, tolerability, and safety were only several weeks in duration. There continues to be a dearth of studies evaluating long-term use of opioids for chronic pain.

Fast Fact

There has been a gradual introduction of new analgesics into medical practice including drugs such as ketamine, gabapentin, pregabalin, and clonidine.

The continued use of opioids in patients with chronic pain may only be contributing to further opioid tolerance, dependency, and adverse effects while adding little to nociception. Opioid-sparing drugs may provide more effective and more specific pain management and reduce the burden of chronic opioid use and adverse effects.

> **Fast Fact**
>
> *The most recent guideline on the use of medications in the treatment of opioid addiction from the American Society of Addiction Medicine (2015) provides only one brief mention of medical cannabis and provides no guidance on the use of cannabinoid medications on the subject.*

TRADITIONAL OPIOID-SPARING MEDICATIONS

There are several classes of drugs that have traditionally been used alone or in combination to reduce opioid use. In addition, nonpharmacologic treatments (e.g., cryotherapy, distraction techniques, breathing and relaxation, acupuncture) supplement pharmacologic analgesics and can be safe and easy to implement.

Acetaminophen

Acetaminophen is the most commonly used nonopioid pain reliever.

Nonsteroidal Anti-Inflammatory Drugs

A wide variety of first- and second-line oral nonsteroidal anti-inflammatory drugs (NSAIDs) are effective for pain relief through anti-inflammatory effects. A study of diclofenac or celecoxib (400 mg loading, 200 mg twice daily) revealed a statistically significant reduction in need of rescue opioid medication during 0 to 24 hours and >24 to 48 hours following bunionectomy compared with placebo.

A study of the NSAID rofecoxib (ROF) found that in acute pain, a single dose of ROF was at least as effective but required less additional opioid analgesia than a single dose of oxycodone/acetaminophen over 6 hours and 24 hours. Over 24 hours, ROF was as effective as the multidose oxycodone/acetaminophen regimen and the use of additional analgesia was similar; however, more adverse events occurred with oxycodone/acetaminophen.

> **Fast Fact**
>
> *The vast majority of opioids prescribed have 325 mg of acetaminophen in combination with the opioid for synergistic effects and need for lower dose of opioid.*

Ketamine

There are active studies for potential use in acute and chronic pain conditions, especially where pain management is difficult with conventional treatments such as opioids.

The principal pharmacologic action of ketamine is the novel effect of N-methyl-d-aspartate (NMDA) receptor antagonism. The NMDA receptor is widely distributed in the central and peripheral nervous systems. It plays a crucial role in the development of severe acute pain and progression to chronic pain—by sustained facilitation of nociceptive transmission.

As an NMDA receptor antagonist, ketamine is expected to reduce or oppose the clinical features of opioid tolerance and opioid-induced hypersensitivity, leading to reduced opioid consumption and improved efficacy of long-term opioids.

Limited clinical evidence available showed that ketamine could neither reduce pain score nor opioid consumption in chronic non-cancer pain patients receiving high-dose opioids.

Fast Fact

The increased use of IV ketamine for acute pain resulted in Consensus Guidelines on the Use of Intravenous Ketamine Infusions for Acute Pain Management From the American Society of Regional Anesthesia and Pain Medicine, the American Academy of Pain Medicine, and the American Society of Anesthesiologists. They recommended acute use of ketamine in emergency situations and the perioperative period for individuals with refractory pain, and in opioid-tolerant patients.

Gabapentin and Pregabalin

Effective for acute and chronic neuropathic pain, several clinical reports suggest the usefulness of gabapentin as analgesic in the treatment of several neuropathic pain syndromes.

In a study where gabapentin was administered as therapy to 22 patients with neuropathic cancer pain that was only partially responsive to opioid therapy:

- Gabapentin was given for at least a week and efficacy was assessed after 7 to 14 days of therapy.
- Global pain score decreased from a mean of 6.4 to 3.2.
- Burning pain intensity decreased from a mean of 5.1 to 2.0.
- Episodes of shooting pain decreased in frequency from 7.2 to 2.2 daily episodes.
- Allodynia was found in nine patients and disappeared in seven during gabapentin administration.

Alpha2 Adrenergic Agonists

Alpha2-adrenoceptor agonists, such as clonidine, are potent analgesic drugs and their analgesic effects can synergize when coadministered. Alpha2-adrenoceptors have potent spinal and systemic analgesic effects.

These supra-additive interactions are potentially beneficial clinically by increasing efficacy and/or reducing the total dose of opioid required to produce sufficient pain relief, and undesired side effects can be minimized. These effects have been shown to occur with both acute and chronic pain in animal models.

Topical Therapies

Topical NSAIDs, anesthetics such as lidocaine, and counterirritants such as camphor, menthol, and capsaicin bypass systemic absorption and achieve efficacy at a low dose by directly delivering the drug to specific injury site. They provide maximum local absorption through the intact skin for the drug to have an effect on acute pain.

Topical NSAIDs of different types and formulations are available both over-the-counter and by prescription.

The use of topical NSAIDs may provide an alternative or complementary approach to oral therapies for treatment of acute musculoskeletal pain with modest adverse effects.

Dronabinol

Dronabinol is currently undergoing a 12-week trial named Dronabinol Opioid Sparing Evaluation (DOSE) to look at these and other harm-reduction effects of coadministered dronabinol and opioids.

- The DOSE trial was scheduled to be completed in July 2019.
- The results have not yet been reported.
- Primary objective of adding cannabinoid medications to chronic opioid therapy is to reduce morbidity and mortality associated with opioids and improve pain and function.
- This should be done while also preventing development of significant adverse cannabinoid effects such as euphoria, psychosis, anxiety, or cannabis dependency.

CANNABINOID MEDICATIONS FOR OPIOID SPARING

Among the over 3 million patients in the United States who use medical cannabis in states with legal medical marijuana programs, chronic pain is by far the most common condition for which medical cannabis is recommended.

The significant legal restrictions associated with medical cannabis being a Schedule I drug and limited availability of effective cannabinoid medications has frustrated attempts to research the efficacy of cannabinoid medications for opioid sparing. However, cannabinoids, when coadministered with opioids, may enable reduced opioid doses without loss of analgesic efficacy.

- Cannabinoids have therapeutic effects on pain via the ECS through allosteric mechanisms on MOR.
- Tetrahydrocannabinol (THC) has beneficial effects on nociceptive pain and neuropathic pain via CB1, and inflammation via CB2 receptor agonism.
- Cannabinoids, via 5HT1a agonism, can have a positive effect on the psychological effects, such as anxiety and depression, caused by chronic pain.

Cannabis sativa contains over a hundred phytocannabinoids, but only THC and cannabidiol (CBD) have been studied extensively. THC has been shown to have 20 times the anti-inflammatory potency of aspirin and twice that of hydrocortisone in neuropathic pain. However, unlike NSAIDs and aspirin, THC does not demonstrate cyclooxygenase (COX) inhibition. COX-1 and COX-2 inhibition are associated with the gastrointestinal and cardiovascular adverse effects associated with NSAIDs.

Fast Fact

Beta caryophyllene, a terpene present in high amounts in some strains of C. sativa, is a CB2 agonist, and greatly increases the synergistic entourage effect for chronic pain and inflammation.

CBD has minimal agonism on ECS receptors but works by increasing the amount of the naturally occurring endocannabinoid, anandamide (AEA), by inhibiting fatty acid amidohydrolase (FAAH). FAAH is the primary hydrolytic enzyme of AEA. CBD impacts CB2 receptors on immune system cells in the brain and body, resulting in pain-relieving anti-inflammatory effects. CBD also has effects independent of the ECS via agonism of 5HT1a receptors and increases in glutamate.

STUDIES OF CANNABINOID AND OPIOID SPARING

A 2017 systematic review of the research using case studies and controlled trials or preclinical and clinical studies was conducted.

- Meta-analysis of preclinical studies indicated that the median effective dose of morphine administered in combination with THC is 3.6 times lower than that of morphine alone.
- The median effective dose for codeine administered in combination with THC was 9.5 times lower than that of codeine alone.
- Large controlled clinical studies showed some clinical benefits of cannabinoids; however, opioid dose changes were rarely reported and mixed findings were observed for analgesia.

Twenty-eight studies provided data relating to the potential opioid-sparing effect of cannabinoids in the context of opioid analgesia.

- Most of the preclinical studies examined reported reduced opioid requirements when coadministered with cannabinoids.
- Few controlled clinical studies measured opioid sparing as an endpoint, and findings relating to analgesia were mixed.
- Two controlled studies found no effect of cannabinoids on opioid dose requirements.
- One case series provided very low-quality evidence of a reduction in opioid dose requirements with cannabinoid coadministration.

OTHER OPIOID-SPARING MEDICATIONS THAT WORK VIA THE ECS

Acetaminophen is one of the most commonly used over-the-counter pain medications. Unlike NSAIDs and aspirin, which are COX inhibitors, acetaminophen is not a COX inhibitor and has no gastrointestinal adverse effects or untoward cardiorenal effects. It is a common opioid-sparing ingredient combined with opioids in most of the common opioid tablets. The previous 500 mg dose of acetaminophen in these combination tablets was reduced to 325 mg to reduce the chance of hepatotoxicity from taking multiple tablets a day.

> **Fast Fact**
>
> *Acetaminophen's mechanism of action has been elusive in the 100 years that it has been in use. However, over the past decade, several studies have confirmed its mechanism of action as a prodrug.*

The metabolite, para-aminophenol, is actually a CB1 selective cannabinoid. It produces analgesia through the indirect agonism of CB1 receptors in the brain and transient receptor potential cation channel subfamily V member 1 (TRPV-1) agonism. Para-aminophenol is also an inhibitor of AEA uptake, leading to increased levels of this endocannabinoid and increased cannabinoid receptor agonism.

The acetaminophen metabolite para-aminophenol is an agonist of the TRPV1 receptor, also known as the capsaicin receptor. TRPV1 is involved with providing the nociceptive sensation of heat and pain. Acetaminophen has analgesic effects through this pathway as well.

Capsaicin is a common ingredient of topical analgesic preparations. It is also a TRPV1 agonist and works by prolonged topical application leading to alleviation of pain via desensitization of TRPV1-mediated release of inflammatory molecules following noxious stimuli.

Bibliography

Argoff, C., McCarberg, B., Gudin, J., Nalamachu, S., & Young, C. (2019). Solu-Matrix® Diclofenac: Sustained opioid-sparing effects in a phase 3 study in patients with postoperative pain. *Pain Medicine, 17*(10), 1933–1941. doi:10.1093/pm/pnw012

Bergamaschi, M. M., Queiroz, R. H., Chagas, M. H., de Oliveira, D. C., De Martinis, B. S., Kapczinski, F., … Crippa, J. A. (2011). Cannabidiol reduces the anxiety induced by simulated public speaking in treatment-naïve social phobia patients. *Neuropsychopharmacology, 36*(6), 1219–1226. doi:10.1038/npp.2011.6

Bicket, M. C., White, E., Pronovost, P. J., Wu, C. L., Yaster, M., & Alexander, G. C. (2019). Opioid oversupply after joint and spine surgery: A prospective cohort study. *Anesthesia and Analgesia, 128*(2), 358–364. doi:10.1213/ANE.0000000000003364

Caraceni, A., Zecca, E., Martini, C., & De Conno, F. (1999). Gabapentin as an adjuvant to opioid analgesia for neuropathic cancer pain. *Journal of Pain and Symptom Management, 17*(6), 441–445. doi:10.1016/s0885-3924(99)00033-0

Chabot-Doré, A. J., Schuster, D. J., Stone, L. S., & Wilcox, G. L. (2015). Analgesic synergy between opioid and α2-adrenoceptors. *British Journal of Pharmacology, 172*(2), 388–402. doi:10.1111/bph.12695

Chou, R., Fanciullo, G. J., Fine, P. G., Adler, J. A., Ballantyne, J. C., Davies, P., … Miaskowski, C. (2009). Clinical guidelines for the use of chronic opioid therapy in chronic noncancer pain. *The Journal of Pain, 10*(2), 113–130. doi:10.1016/j.jpain.2008.10.008

de Mello Schier, A. R., de Oliveira Ribeiro, N. P., Coutinho, D. S., Machado, S., Arias-Carrión, O., Crippa, J. A., … Silva, A. C. (2014). Antidepressant-like and anxiolytic-like effects of cannabidiol: A chemical compound of Cannabis sativa. *CNS Neurological Disorders Drug Targets, 13*(6), 953–960.

Desjardins, P., Bird, S., Petruschke, R., & Chang, D. (2004). NSAIDs and acetaminophen: Comparison of opioid rescue use between Rofecoxib and Oxycodone/Acetaminophen in a double-blind, randomized trial of patients with acute pain. *The Journal of Pain, 5*(3), S64. doi:10.1016/j.jpain.2004.02.222

Gatti, A., Sabato, E., Di Paolo, A. R., Mammucari, M., & Sabato, A. F. (2010). Oxycodone/paracetamol: A low-dose synergic combination useful in different types of pain. *Clinical Drug Investigation, 30*(Suppl. 2), 3–14. doi:10.2165/1158414-S0-000000000-00000

Gorzalka, B. B., Hill, M. N., & Hillard, C. J. (2008). Regulation of endocannabinoid signaling by stress: Implications for stress-related affective disorders. *Neuroscience & Biobehavioral Reviews, 32*(6), 1152–1160. doi:10.1016/j.neubiorev.2008.03.004

Kapural, L., Kapural, M., Bensitel, T., & Sessler, D. I. (2010). Opioid-sparing effect of intravenous outpatient ketamine infusions appears short-lived in chronic-pain patients with high opioid requirements. *Pain Physician, 13*(4), 389–394.

Mellick, G. A., Mellicy, L. B., & Mellick, L. B. (1995). Gabapentin in the management of reflex sympathetic dystrophy. *Journal of Pain and Symptom Management, 10*(4), 265–266. doi:10.1016/0885-3924(95)00001-F

Narang, S., Gibson, D., Wasan, A. D., Ross, E. L., Michna, E., Nedeljkovic, S. S., & Jamison, R. N. (2008). Efficacy of dronabinol as an adjuvant treatment for chronic pain patients on opioid therapy. *The Journal of Pain, 9*(3), 254–264. doi:10.1016/j.jpain.2007.10.018

Nielsen, S., Sabioni, P., Trigo, J. M., Ware, M. A., Betz-Stablein, B. D., Murnion, B., ... Le Foll, B. (2017). Opioid-sparing effect of cannabinoids: A systematic review and meta-analysis. *Neuropsychopharmacology, 42*(9), 1752–1765. doi:10.1038/npp.2017.51

Peng, P. W., Wijeysundera, D. N., & Li, C. C. (2007). Use of gabapentin for perioperative pain control—A meta-analysis. *Pain Research and Management, 12*(2), 85–92. doi:10.1155/2007/840572

Rousseau, A. F., Lecoq, J. P., Carlier, A., Deleuze, J. P., Dubuisson, A., Lamy, M., & Franssen, C. (2006). Opioids sparing effect of gabapentin in neurogenic thoracic outlet syndrome surgery. *European Journal of Anaesthesiology, 23*, 223.

Russo, E. B. (2008). Cannabinoids in the management of difficult to treat pain. *Therapeutics and Clinical Risk Management, 4*(1), 245–259. doi:10.2147/tcrm.s1928

Schwenk, E. S., Viscusi, E. R., Buvanendran, A., Hurley, R. W., Wasan, A. D., Narouze, S., ... Cohen, S. P. (2018). Consensus guidelines on the use of intravenous ketamine infusions for acute pain management from the American Society of Regional Anesthesia and Pain Medicine, the American Academy of Pain Medicine, and the American Society of Anesthesiologists. *Regional Anesthesia and Pain Medicine, 43*(5), 456–466. doi:10.1097/AAP.0000000000000806

Sommer, C., Welsch, P., Klose, P., Schaefert, R., Petzke, F., & Häuser, W. (2015). [Opioids in chronic neuropathic pain. A systematic review and meta-analysis of efficacy, tolerability and safety in randomized placebo-controlled studies of at least 4 weeks duration]. *Schmerz, 29*(1), 35–46. doi:10.1007/s00482-014-1455-x

Sullivan, D., Lyons, M., Montgomery, R., & Quinlan-Colwell, A. (2016). Exploring opioid-sparing multimodal analgesia options in trauma: A nursing perspective. *Journal of Trauma Nursing, 23*(6), 361–375. doi:10.1097/JTN.0000000000000250

Tajerian, M., Millecamps, M., & Stone, L. S. (2012). Morphine and clonidine synergize to ameliorate low back pain in mice. *Pain Research and Treatment, 2012*, 150842. doi:10.1155/2012/150842

Tsui, P., & Che, M. C. (2017). Ketamine: An old drug revitalized in pain medicine. *BJA Education, 17*(3), 84–87. doi:10.1093/bjaed/mkw034

Wang, W., Sun, D., Pan, B., Roberts, C. J., Sun, X., Hillard, C. J., & Liu, Q. S. (2010). Deficiency in endocannabinoid signaling in the nucleus accumbens induced by chronic unpredictable stress. *Neuropsychopharmacology, 35*(11), 2249–2261. doi:10.1038/npp.2010.99

Appendices

Appendix A

CENTERS FOR DISEASE CONTROL AND PREVENTION GUIDELINE FOR PRESCRIBING OPIOIDS FOR CHRONIC PAIN

IMPROVING PRACTICE THROUGH RECOMMENDATIONS

CDC's *Guideline for Prescribing Opioids for Chronic Pain* is intended to improve communication between providers and patients about the risks and benefits of opioid therapy for chronic pain, improve the safety and effectiveness of pain treatment, and reduce the risks associated with long-term opioid therapy, including opioid use disorder and overdose. The Guideline is not intended for patients who are in active cancer treatment, palliative care, or end-of-life care.

DETERMINING WHEN TO INITIATE OR CONTINUE OPIOIDS FOR CHRONIC PAIN

1. Nonpharmacologic therapy and nonopioid pharmacologic therapy are preferred for chronic pain. Clinicians should consider opioid therapy only if expected benefits for both pain and function are anticipated to outweigh risks to the patient. If opioids are used, they should be combined with nonpharmacologic therapy and nonopioid pharmacologic therapy, as appropriate.

2. Before starting opioid therapy for chronic pain, clinicians should establish treatment goals with all patients, including realistic goals for pain and function, and should consider how opioid therapy will be discontinued if benefits do not outweigh risks. Clinicians should continue opioid therapy only if there is clinically meaningful improvement in pain and function that outweighs risks to patient safety.

3. Before starting and periodically during opioid therapy, clinicians should discuss with patients known risks and realistic benefits of opioid therapy and patient and clinician responsibilities for managing therapy.

CLINICAL REMINDERS

- Opioids are not first-line or routine therapy for chronic pain
- Establish and measure goals for pain and function
- Discuss benefits and risks and availability of nonopioid therapies with patient

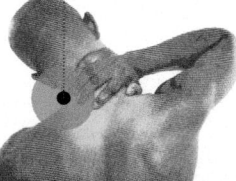

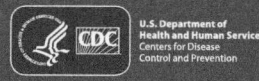

U.S. Department of Health and Human Services
Centers for Disease Control and Prevention

LEARN MORE | www.cdc.gov/drugoverdose/prescribing/guideline.html

OPIOID SELECTION, DOSAGE, DURATION, FOLLOW-UP, AND DISCONTINUATION

CLINICAL REMINDERS

- Use immediate-release opioids when starting
- Start low and go slow
- When opioids are needed for acute pain, prescribe no more than needed
- Do not prescribe ER/LA opioids for acute pain
- Follow-up and re-evaluate risk of harm; reduce dose or taper and discontinue if needed

4. When starting opioid therapy for chronic pain, clinicians should prescribe immediate-release opioids instead of extended-release/long-acting (ER/LA) opioids.

5. When opioids are started, clinicians should prescribe the lowest effective dosage. Clinicians should use caution when prescribing opioids at any dosage, should carefully reassess evidence of individual benefits and risks when considering increasing dosage to ≥50 morphine milligram equivalents (MME)/day, and should avoid increasing dosage to ≥90 MME/day or carefully justify a decision to titrate dosage to ≥90 MME/day.

6. Long-term opioid use often begins with treatment of acute pain. When opioids are used for acute pain, clinicians should prescribe the lowest effective dose of immediate-release opioids and should prescribe no greater quantity than needed for the expected duration of pain severe enough to require opioids. Three days or less will often be sufficient; more than seven days will rarely be needed.

7. Clinicians should evaluate benefits and harms with patients within 1 to 4 weeks of starting opioid therapy for chronic pain or of dose escalation. Clinicians should evaluate benefits and harms of continued therapy with patients every 3 months or more frequently. If benefits do not outweigh harms of continued opioid therapy, clinicians should optimize other therapies and work with patients to taper opioids to lower dosages or to taper and discontinue opioids.

ASSESSING RISK AND ADDRESSING HARMS OF OPIOID USE

8. Before starting and periodically during continuation of opioid therapy, clinicians should evaluate risk factors for opioid-related harms. Clinicians should incorporate into the management plan strategies to mitigate risk, including considering offering naloxone when factors that increase risk for opioid overdose, such as history of overdose, history of substance use disorder, higher opioid dosages (≥50 MME/day), or concurrent benzodiazepine use, are present.

9. Clinicians should review the patient's history of controlled substance prescriptions using state prescription drug monitoring program (PDMP) data to determine whether the patient is receiving opioid dosages or dangerous combinations that put him or her at high risk for overdose. Clinicians should review PDMP data when starting opioid therapy for chronic pain and periodically during opioid therapy for chronic pain, ranging from every prescription to every 3 months.

10. When prescribing opioids for chronic pain, clinicians should use urine drug testing before starting opioid therapy and consider urine drug testing at least annually to assess for prescribed medications as well as other controlled prescription drugs and illicit drugs.

11. Clinicians should avoid prescribing opioid pain medication and benzodiazepines concurrently whenever possible.

12. Clinicians should offer or arrange evidence-based treatment (usually medication-assisted treatment with buprenorphine or methadone in combination with behavioral therapies) for patients with opioid use disorder.

CLINICAL REMINDERS

- Evaluate risk factors for opioid-related harms
- Check PDMP for high dosages and prescriptions from other providers
- Use urine drug testing to identify prescribed substances and undisclosed use
- Avoid concurrent benzodiazepine and opioid prescribing
- Arrange treatment for opioid use disorder if needed

LEARN MORE | www.cdc.gov/drugoverdose/prescribing/guideline.html

Appendix B

NATIONAL INSTITUTES OF DRUG ABUSE QUICK SCREEN AND NIDA-MODIFIED ASSIST SCREENINGS FOR OPIOID USE DISORDER

Name: .... Sex ( ) F ( ) M Age.......
Interviewer... Date ....../....../......
Introduction (Please read to patient)

Hi, I'm_____, nice to meet you. If it's okay with you, I'd like to ask you a few questions that will help me give you better medical care. The questions relate to your experience with alcohol, cigarettes, and other drugs. Some of the substances we'll talk about are prescribed by a doctor (such as pain medications). But I will only record those if you have taken them for reasons or in doses <u>other than prescribed</u>. I'll also ask you about illicit or illegal drug use––but only to better diagnose and treat you.

---

[1] *This guide is designed to assist clinicians serving adult patients in screening for drug use. The NIDA Quick Screen was adapted from the single-question screen for drug use in primary care by Saitz et al. (available at* http://archinte.ama-assn.org/cgi/reprint/170/13/1155) *and the National Institute on Alcohol Abuse and Alcoholism's screening question on heavy drinking days (available at* http://pubs.niaaa.nih.gov/publications/Practitioner/CliniciansGuide2005/clinicians_guide.htm). *The NIDA-modified ASSIST was adapted from the World Health Organization (WHO) Alcohol, Smoking, and Substance Involvement Screening Test (ASSIST), Version 3.0, developed and published by WHO (available at* http://www.who.int/substance_abuse/activities/assist_v3_english.pdf).

NIDA *Quick Screen* Question: In the past year, how often have you used the following?	Never	Once or Twice	Monthly	Weekly	Daily or Almost Daily
Alcohol ■ **For men, 5 or more drinks a day** ■ **For women, 4 or more drinks a day**					
Tobacco Products					
Prescription Drugs for Nonmedical Reasons					
Illegal Drugs					

Instructions: For each substance, mark in the appropriate column. For example, if the patient has used cocaine monthly in the past year, mark the "Monthly" column in the "illegal drug" row.

- If the patient says **"NO"** for all drugs in the Quick Screen, reinforce abstinence. **Screening is complete.**
- If the patient says **"Yes"** to **one or more days of heavy drinking**, *patient is an at-risk drinker*. Please see NIAAA website "How to Help Patients Who Drink Too Much: A Clinical Approach" http://pubs.niaaa.nih.gov/publications/Practitioner/CliniciansGuide2005/clinicians_guide.htm, for information to **Assess, Advise, Assist, and Arrange** help for at-risk drinkers or patients with alcohol use disorders.
- If patient says **"Yes"** to **use of tobacco:** *Any* current tobacco use places a patient at risk. Advise *all tobacco users to quit*. For more information on smoking cessation, please see "Helping Smokers Quit: A Guide for Clinicians" http://www.ahrq.gov/clinic/tobacco/clinhlpsmksqt.htm
- If the patient says **"Yes"** to **use of illegal drugs or prescription drugs for nonmedical reasons**, proceed to **Question 1** of the NIDA-Modified ASSIST.

QUESTIONS 1 TO 8 OF THE NIDA-MODIFIED ASSIST V2.0

Instructions: Patients may fill in the following form themselves, but screening personnel should offer to read the questions aloud in a private setting and complete the form for the patient. To preserve confidentiality, a protective sheet should be placed on top of the questionnaire so it will not be seen by other patients after it is completed but before it is filed in the medical record.

Question 1 of 8, NIDA-Modified ASSIST Yes No

In your *LIFETIME*, which of the following substances have you ever used?

*Note for Physicians: For prescription medications, please report nonmedical use only.

a. **Cannabis** (marijuana, pot, grass, hash, etc.)

b. **Cocaine** (coke, crack, etc.)

c. **Prescription stimulants** (Ritalin, Concerta, Dexedrine, Adderall, diet pills, etc.)

d. **Methamphetamine** (speed, crystal meth, ice, etc.)

e. **Inhalants** (nitrous oxide, glue, gas, paint thinner, etc.)

f. **Sedatives or sleeping pills** (Valium, Serepax, Ativan, Xanax, Librium, Rohypnol, GHB, etc.)

g. **Hallucinogens** (LSD, acid, mushrooms, PCP, Special K, ecstasy, etc.)

h. **Street opioids** (heroin, opium, etc.)

i. **Prescription opioids** (fentanyl, oxycodone [OxyContin, Percocet], hydrocodone [Vicodin], methadone, buprenorphine, etc.)

j. **Other—specify:**

- Given the patient's response to the Quick Screen, the patient *should* not indicate **"NO"** for all drugs in Question 1. If they do, remind them that their answers to the Quick Screen indicate they used an illegal or prescription drug for nonmedical reasons within the past year and then **repeat Question 1**. If the patient indicates that the drug used is not listed, please mark **"Yes"** next to "Other" and continue to **Question 2** of the NIDA-Modified ASSIST.

Question 2 of 8, NIDA-Modified ASSIST

2. In the past three months, how often have you used the substances you mentioned (first drug, second drug, etc.)?	Never	Once or Twice	Monthly	Weekly	Daily or Almost Daily
■ Cannabis (marijuana, pot, grass, hash, etc.)	0	2	3	4	6
■ Cocaine (coke, crack, etc.)	0	2	3	4	6
■ Prescription stimulants (Ritalin, Concerta, Dexedrine, Adderall, diet pills, etc.)	0	2	3	4	6
■ Methamphetamine (speed, crystal meth, ice, etc.)	0	2	3	4	6
■ Inhalants (nitrous oxide, glue, gas, paint thinner, etc.)	0	2	3	4	6
■ Sedatives or sleeping pills (Valium, Serepax, Ativan, Librium, Xanax, Rohypnol, GHB, etc.)	0	2	3	4	6
■ Hallucinogens (LSD, acid, mushrooms, PCP, Special K, ecstasy, etc.)	0	2	3	4	6
■ Street opioids (heroin, opium, etc.)	0	2	3	4	6
■ Prescription opioids (fentanyl, oxycodone [OxyContin, Percocet], hydrocodone [Vicodin], methadone, buprenorphine, etc.)	0	2	3	4	6
■ Other—Specify:	0	2	3	4	6

- If the patient says **"Yes"** to any of the drugs, proceed to **Question 2** of the NIDA-Modified ASSIST.
- For patients who report **"Never"** having used any drug in the past 3 months: **Go to Questions 6–8**.
- For any recent **illicit or nonmedical prescription drug use**, go to **Question 3**.

3. <u>In the past 3 months</u>, how often have you had a strong desire or urge to use the first drug, second drug, etc.?	Never	Once or Twice	Monthly	Weekly	Daily or Almost Daily
a. Cannabis (marijuana, pot, grass, hash, etc.)	0	3	4	5	6
b. Cocaine (coke, crack, etc.)	0	3	4	5	6
c. Prescribed Amphetamine type stimulants (Ritalin, Concerta, Dexedrine, Adderall, diet pills, etc.)	0	3	4	5	6
d. Methamphetamine (speed, crystal meth, ice, etc.)	0	3	4	5	6
e. Inhalants (nitrous oxide, glue, gas, paint thinner, etc.)	0	3	4	5	6
f. Sedatives or sleeping pills (Valium, Serepax, Ativan, Librium, Xanax, Rohypnol, GHB, etc.)	0	3	4	5	6
g. Hallucinogens (LSD, acid, mushrooms, PCP, Special K, ecstasy, etc.)	0	3	4	5	6
h. Street Opioids (heroin, opium, etc.)	0	3	4	5	6
i. Prescribed opioids (fentanyl, oxycodone [OxyContin, Percocet], hydrocodone [Vicodin], methadone, buprenorphine, etc.)	0	3	4	5	6
j. Other—Specify:	0	3	4	5	6

4. During the past 3 months, how often has your use of the first drug, second drug, etc. led to health, social, legal, or financial problems?	Never	Once or Twice	Monthly	Weekly	Daily or Almost Daily
a. Cannabis (marijuana, pot, grass, hash, etc.)	0	4	5	6	7
b. Cocaine (coke, crack, etc.)	0	4	5	6	7
c. Prescribed Amphetamine type stimulants (Ritalin, Concerta, Dexedrine, Adderall, diet pills, etc.)	0	4	5	6	7
d. Methamphetamine (speed, crystal meth, ice, etc.)	0	4	5	6	7
e. Inhalants (nitrous oxide, glue, gas, paint thinner, etc.)	0	4	5	6	7
f. Sedatives or sleeping pills (Valium, Serepax, Ativan, Librium, Xanax, Rohypnol, GHB, etc.)	0	4	5	6	7
g. Hallucinogens (LSD, acid, mushrooms, PCP, Special K, ecstasy, etc.)	0	4	5	6	7
h. Street opioids (heroin, opium, etc.)	0	4	5	6	7
i. Prescribed opioids (fentanyl, oxycodone [OxyContin, Percocet], hydrocodone [Vicodin], methadone, buprenorphine, etc.)	0	4	5	6	7
j. Other—Specify:	0	4	5	6	7

5. During the past 3 months, how often have you failed to do what was normally expected of you because of your use of the first drug, second drug, etc.?	Never	Once or Twice	Monthly	Weekly	Daily or Almost Daily
a. Cannabis (marijuana, pot, grass, hash, etc.)	0	5	6	7	8
b. Cocaine (coke, crack, etc.)	0	5	6	7	8
c. Prescribed Amphetamine type stimulants (Ritalin, Concerta, Dexedrine, Adderall, diet pills, etc.)	0	5	6	7	8
d. Methamphetamine (speed, crystal meth, ice, etc.)	0	5	6	7	8
e. Inhalants (nitrous oxide, glue, gas, paint thinner, etc.)	0	5	6	7	8
f. Sedatives or sleeping pills (Valium, Serepax, Ativan, Librium, Xanax, Rohypnol, GHB, etc.)	0	5	6	7	8
g. Hallucinogens (LSD, acid, mushrooms, PCP, Special K, ecstasy, etc.)	0	5	6	7	8
h. Street Opioids (heroin, opium, etc.)	0	5	6	7	8
i. Prescribed opioids (fentanyl, oxycodone [OxyContin, Percocet], hydrocodone [Vicodin], methadone, buprenorphine, etc.)	0	5	6	7	8
j. Other—Specify:	0	5	6	7	8

Instructions: Ask Questions 6 and 7 for all substances <u>ever used</u> (i.e., those endorsed in Question 1).

6. Has a friend or relative or anyone else <u>ever</u> expressed concern about your use of the first drug, second drug, etc.?	No, never	Yes, but not in the past 3 months	Yes, in the past 3 months
a. Cannabis (marijuana, pot, grass, hash, etc.)	0	3	6
b. Cocaine (coke, crack, etc.)	0	3	6
c. Prescribed Amphetamine type stimulants (Ritalin, Concerta, Dexedrine, Adderall, diet pills, etc.)	0	3	6
d. Methamphetamine (speed, crystal meth, ice, etc.)	0	3	6
e. Inhalants (nitrous oxide, glue, gas, paint thinner, etc.)	0	3	6
f. Sedatives or sleeping pills (Valium, Serepax, Xanax, Ativan, Librium, Rohypnol, GHB, etc.)	0	3	6
g. Hallucinogens (LSD, acid, mushrooms, PCP, Special K, ecstasy, etc.)	0	3	6
h. Street opioids (heroin, opium, etc.)	0	3	6
i. Prescribed opioids (fentanyl, oxycodone [OxyContin, Percocet], hydrocodone [Vicodin], methadone, buprenorphine, etc.)	0	3	6
j. Other—Specify:	0	3	6

7. Have you ever tried and failed to control, cut down or stop using the first drug, second drug, etc.?	No, never	Yes, but not in the past 3 months	Yes, in the past 3 months
a. Cannabis (marijuana, pot, grass, hash, etc.)	0	3	6
b. Cocaine (coke, crack, etc.)	0	3	6
c. Prescribed Amphetamine type stimulants (Ritalin, Concerta, Dexedrine, Adderall, diet pills, etc.)	0	3	6
d. Methamphetamine (speed, crystal meth, ice, etc.)	0	3	6
e. Inhalants (nitrous oxide, glue, gas, paint thinner, etc.)	0	3	6
f. Sedatives or sleeping pills (Valium, Serepax, Xanax, Ativan, Librium, Rohypnol, GHB, etc.)	0	3	6
g. Hallucinogens (LSD, acid, mushrooms, PCP, Special K, ecstasy, etc.)	0	3	6
h. Street opioids (heroin, opium, etc.)	0	3	6
i. Prescribed opioids (fentanyl, oxycodone [OxyContin, Percocet], hydrocodone [Vicodin], methadone, buprenorphine, etc.)	0	3	6
j. Other—Specify:	0	3	6

Instructions: Ask Question 8 if the patient endorses any drug that might be injected, including those that might be listed in the other category (e.g., steroids). <u>Circle appropriate response</u>.

8. Have you ever used any drug by injection (NONMEDICAL USE ONLY)?	No, never	Yes, but not in the past 3 months	Yes, in the past 3 months

- Recommend to patients reporting any prior or current intravenous drug use that they get tested for HIV and hepatitis B/C.
- If patient reports using a drug by injection in the past three months, ask about their pattern of injecting during this period to determine their risk levels and the best course of intervention.
  - If patient responds that they inject once weekly or less or fewer than 3 days in a row, provide a brief intervention including a discussion of the risks associated with injecting.
  - If patient responds that they inject more than once per week or 3 or more days in a row, refer for further assessment.

Note: Recommend to patients reporting any current use of alcohol or illicit drugs that they get tested for HIV and other sexually transmitted diseases.

Tally Sheet for Scoring the Full NIDA-Modified ASSIST

Instructions: For each substance (labeled a–j), add up the scores received for abovementioned questions 2–7. This is the Substance Involvement (SI) score. Do not include the results from either the Q1 or Q8 (above) in your SI scores.

Substance Involvement Score	Total (SI SCORE)
a. Cannabis (marijuana, pot, grass, hash, etc.)	
b. Cocaine (coke, crack, etc.)	
c. Prescription stimulants (Ritalin, Concerta, Dexedrine, Adderall, diet pills, etc.)	
d. Methamphetamine (speed, crystal meth, ice, etc.)	
e. Inhalants (nitrous oxide, glue, gas, paint thinner, etc.)	
f. Sedatives or sleeping pills (Valium, Serepax, Xanax, Ativan, Librium, Rohypnol, GHB, etc.)	
g. Hallucinogens (LSD, acid, mushrooms, PCP, Special K, ecstasy, etc.)	
h. Street Opioids (heroin, opium, etc.)	
i. Prescription opioids (fentanyl, oxycodone [OxyContin, Percocet], hydrocodone [Vicodin], methadone, buprenorphine, etc.)	
j. Other—Specify:	

Use the Resultant SI Score to identify patient's risk level.

To determine patient's Hrisk level H based on his or her HSI scoreH, see the following table:

Level of risk associated with different Substance Involvement Score ranges for Illicit or nonmedical prescription drug use	
0–3	Lower risk
4–26	Moderate risk
27+	High risk

Appendix C

CENTERS FOR DISEASE CONTROL AND PREVENTION CALCULATING TOTAL DAILY DOSE OF OPIOIDS FOR SAFER DOSAGE

Higher Dosage, Higher Risk.

Higher dosages of opioids are associated with higher risk of overdose and death—even relatively low dosages (20-50 morphine milligram equivalents (MME) per day) increase risk. Higher dosages haven't been shown to reduce pain over the long term. One randomized trial found no difference in pain or function between a more liberal opioid dose escalation strategy (with average final dosage 52 MME) and maintenance of current dosage (average final dosage 40 MME).

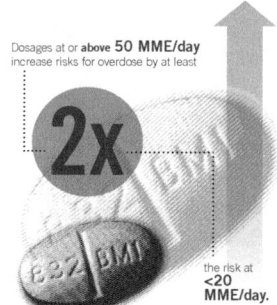

Dosages at or **above 50 MME/day** increase risks for overdose by at least **2x** the risk at **<20 MME/day**.

WHY IS IT IMPORTANT TO CALCULATE THE TOTAL DAILY DOSAGE OF OPIOIDS?

Patients prescribed higher opioid dosages are at higher risk of overdose death.

In a national sample of Veterans Health Administration (VHA) patients with chronic pain receiving opioids from 2004–2009, **patients who died** of opioid overdose were prescribed an average of **98 MME/day**, while **other patients** were prescribed an average of **48 MME/day**.

Calculating the total daily dose of opioids helps identify patients who may benefit from closer monitoring, reduction or tapering of opioids, prescribing of naloxone, or other measures to reduce risk of overdose.

HOW MUCH IS 50 OR 90 MME/DAY FOR COMMONLY PRESCRIBED OPIOIDS?

50 MME/day:
- 50 mg of hydrocodone (10 tablets of hydrocodone/acetaminophen 5/300)
- 33 mg of oxycodone (~2 tablets of oxycodone sustained-release 15 mg)
- 12 mg of methadone (<3 tablets of methadone 5 mg)

90 MME/day:
- 90 mg of hydrocodone (9 tablets of hydrocodone/acetaminophen 10/325)
- 60 mg of oxycodone (~2 tablets of oxycodone sustained-release 30 mg)
- ~20 mg of methadone (4 tablets of methadone 5 mg)

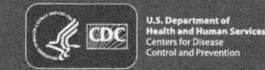

U.S. Department of Health and Human Services
Centers for Disease Control and Prevention

LEARN MORE | www.cdc.gov/drugoverdose/prescribing/guideline.html

HOW SHOULD THE TOTAL DAILY DOSE OF OPIOIDS BE CALCULATED?

1. **DETERMINE** the total daily amount of each opioid the patient takes.
2. **CONVERT** each to MMEs—multiply the dose for each opioid by the conversion factor. (*see table*)
3. **ADD** them together.

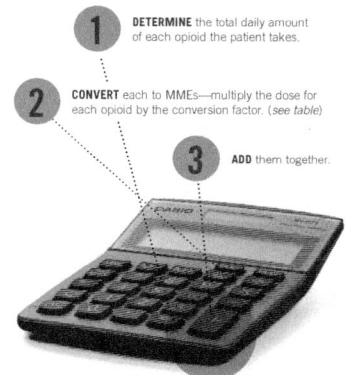

Calculating morphine milligram equivalents (MME)

OPIOID (doses in mg/day except where noted)	CONVERSION FACTOR
Codeine	0.15
Fentanyl transdermal (in mcg/hr)	2.4
Hydrocodone	1
Hydromorphone	4
Methadone	
1-20 mg/day	4
21-40 mg/day	8
41-60 mg/day	10
≥ 61-80 mg/day	12
Morphine	1
Oxycodone	1.5
Oxymorphone	3

These dose conversions are estimated and cannot account for all individual differences in genetics and pharmacokinetics.

CAUTION:
- Do not use the calculated dose in MMEs to determine dosage for converting one opioid to another—the new opioid should be lower to avoid unintentional overdose caused by incomplete cross-tolerance and individual differences in opioid pharmacokinetics. Consult the medication label.

USE EXTRA CAUTION:
- **Methadone:** the conversion factor increases at higher doses
- **Fentanyl:** dosed in mcg/hr instead of mg/day, and absorption is affected by heat and other factors

HOW SHOULD PROVIDERS USE THE TOTAL DAILY OPIOID DOSE IN CLINICAL PRACTICE?

- Use caution when prescribing opioids at any dosage and prescribe the lowest effective dose.
- Use extra precautions when increasing to ≥50 MME per day* such as:
  - Monitor and assess pain and function more frequently.
  - Discuss reducing dose or tapering and discontinuing opioids if benefits do not outweigh harms.
  - Consider offering naloxone.
- Avoid or carefully justify increasing dosage to ≥90 MME/day.*

*These dosage thresholds are based on overdose risk when opioids are prescribed for pain and should not guide dosing of medication-assisted treatment for opioid use disorder.

LEARN MORE | www.cdc.gov/drugoverdose/prescribing/guideline.html

Index

absenteeism, 19
abuse-deterrent opioid formulations (ADFs), 156
acetaminophen, 8, 154, 167, 202, 207
acute pain, 140. *See also* chronic pain
addiction
    cannabis, 133
    definition of, 180
    opioid. *See* opioid epidemic
    rates, illicit drug, 133
ADFs. *See* abuse-deterrent opioid formulations
adolescents, use cannabinoid medications in, 89, 100
AEA. *See* anandamide
2-AG. *See* 2-arachidonoylglycerol
alcohol
    consumption after using cannabis, 131
    interaction of nabiximols with, 99
alpha2-adrenoceptor agonists, 204
alpha-humulene, 82
alpha-pinene, 80, 81
American Academy of Neurology, 171
American College of Obstetrics and Gynecology, 32
American Psychiatric Society, 25
American Society for Addiction Medicine (ASAM), 19
American Society for Pharmacology and Experimental Therapeutics, 193
American Society of Addiction Medicine, 202
analgesics, 76, 201, 202, 207
anandamide (AEA), 58, 59, 60, 64, 66, 73, 95, 180, 205
Anslinger, Harry, 44
antihistamines, 60
anxiety, and chronic pain, 141
anxiety disorders, 29, 30
2-arachidonoylglycerol (2-AG), 58, 59, 64, 66, 73, 180
arthritis, 167
ASAM. *See* American Society for Addiction Medicine
aspirin, 44
Axis I disorders, 29

barbiturates, 44
behavioral therapy, 16, 32
benzodiazepines, 5, 6, 10, 158, 161
beta-caryophyllene, 80, 82, 205
BHO. *See* butane hash oil
biased signaling, in endocannabinoid system, 66
bongs, 114, 115

botanical drugs, *vs.* single molecule drugs, 85
brain
  densest receptor concentrations in, 57
  functions, affected by ECS, 57–58
  reward and motivation system, 27–29
breathing problems, and cannabis use, 127–128
budder, 110, 111, 112
budtenders, 108
buprenorphine, 10, 16, 17, 33, 34, 161
butane hash oil (BHO), 110, 111

camphor, 204
cancer-related pain, chronic, 145
cannabichromene (CBC), 77
cannabicyclol, 77
cannabidiol (CBD) (Epidiolex®), 42, 48, 49, 55, 58, 59, 73, 74–75, 80, 83, 90, 92, 95–98, 120, 122, 168, 169, 171, 172, 183, 196, 205–206
  binding to receptors, 66
  CBD:THC ratio, 84, 172
  mental effects of, 130
  molecular structure of, 75
  non-FDA-approved, safety concerns, 102–103
  and opioid relapse, 188
  and opioid withdrawal, 187
  properties of, 75
  treatment studies, 98
cannabigerol (CBG), 76
cannabinoid hyperemesis syndrome (CHS), 129, 132
cannabinoid medications (CMs), 10, 183. *See also* cannabis
  as adjuncts to opioids, 191–196
  for chronic pain, 165–167, 185, 186
    emotional response, 171–172
    spasms and spasticity, 170–171
    studies, 167–170
  combination with opioids, 184–186, 191–192, 206. *See also* opioid sparing
    afferent spinal cord pain messaging, dampening of, 193
    allosteric modulation of MOR, 193
    emotional response to pain, decrease in, 193
    inflammation, decrease in, 193
    opioid relapse, 187–188
    opioid sparing, 186
    opioid weaning, 187
    opioid withdrawal, 187
    spasms/spasticity, decrease in, 194
    studies, 193–194
  current clinical trials, 101
  FDA-approved, 87–88
  future, 101
  isolate. *See* isolate cannabinoid medications
  isolate vs. whole plant extract dosing curve, 101
  for opioid sparing, 205–206. *See also* opioid sparing
  selection of, 196
  synthetic, 87–93
cannabinoids, 40, 49, 61, 63–64. *See also* endocannabinoid system (ECS); terpenes
  entourage effect, 83
  interaction with ECS receptors, 66
  major, 73–75
  minor, 75–78
  psychoactive/nonpsychoactive effects, guide for, 79
  and retrograde inhibition, 67
cannabinol (CBN), 77, 78
cannabis, 8, 60, 73, 75, 166. *See also* cannabinoid medications (CMs)
  abuse, health effects of, 131–133
  ailments treated using, 44
  as an adjunct to opioids, 191–192
    contrary evidence, 194–195

recent studies, 193–194
concentrates, 110–113, 132
factors that affect reaction to, 125–126
federal legal framework, 48–50
flower, 109–110
interaction with medications, 131
legal considerations for patients, 51–52
medical. *See* medical marijuana
overuse/abuse/addiction, symptoms of, 133
present legal status of, 45–48
research-grade, 48
side effects of. *See* side effects of cannabis use
things to avoid while using, 131
types of, 39–42
US prohibition, 44
use, early history of, 42–44
Cannabis indica, 39, 41, 44
Cannabis ruderalis, 39, 42
Cannabis sativa L., 39, 40, 95, 96, 98, 101, 169, 205
cannflavins, 195
capsaicin, 204, 207
capsaicin receptor, 167, 207
caregiver burden, 20
carfentanyl, 8
CB1 receptor, 59, 64, 95, 96, 99, 154, 180
   binding sites of, 66
   and cannabinoid medications, 167
   distribution in brain, 181
   locations of, 65, 66
   and MORs, 183, 193
   and opioids reward/withdrawal, 184–185
   and synthetic cannabinoid medications, 89, 91, 92
CB2 receptor, 59, 64–65, 95, 99, 180, 192
   and cannabinoid medications, 167, 170
   locations of, 65, 66
CBC. *See* cannabichromene
CBD. *See* cannabidiol (Epidiolex®)
CBG. *See* cannabigerol
CBN. *See* cannabinol
CDC. *See* Centers for Disease Control and Prevention
CDH. *See* chronic daily headache
CEDS. *See* clinical endocannabinoid deficiency syndrome
celecoxib, 202
Center for Medicinal Cannabis Research (CMCR), University of California, 166
Centers for Disease Control and Prevention (CDC), 5, 14
   dosage of opioids, calculation of, 227–228
   Guidelines for Prescribing Opioids for Chronic Pain, 4, 157, 213–214
   opioid treatment recommendations, 157–158
   Prescribing Opioids for Chronic Pain, 8
central nervous system (CNS), 27–28, 61, 100, 143, 144, 167, 180
child development problems during/after pregnancy, 128–129
children
   unintentional pediatric cannabis exposures, 119, 132
   use of cannabinoid medications in, 89, 100
chronic daily headache (CDH), 147
chronic pain, 3–4. *See also* pain
   cannabinoid medications for. *See under* cannabinoid medications (CMs)
   cost of, 140
   definition of, 140
   diagnosis of, 142
   epidemic, 5
   epidemiology of, 139–140
   opioid sparing for, 201–202
   opioids for, 201

chronic pain (*cont.*)
  CDC treatment recommendations, 157–158
  noncancer chronic pain, current guidelines, 153
  scientific evidence, 154
  primary pain syndromes, 142–145
  as qualifying condition, 185
  risk factors for developing, 141–142
  secondary pain syndromes, 142, 145–148
  treatment costs. *See* costs of opioid epidemic
chronic postsurgical/posttraumatic pain, 145
CHS. *See* cannabinoid hyperemesis syndrome
clinical endocannabinoid deficiency syndrome (CEDS), 143, 170
clonidine, 34, 201, 204
CMCR. *See* Center for Medicinal Cannabis Research, University of California
CMs. *See* cannabinoid medications
CNS. *See* central nervous system
codeine, 206
cognitive and behavioral therapy, 33
Cole Memos (2011–2014), 48–49
COMM. *See* current opioid misuse measure
complex regional pain syndrome (CRPS), 142, 143–144
Conant v. Walters, 50
concentrates, cannabis, 110–113, 132
condition place preference (CPP), 183
conduction vaporizers, 115
Controlled Substances Act (CSA), 45, 47, 48, 90, 92, 102
convection vaporizers, 115
costs of opioid epidemic, 13–14
  adverse effects treatment, 20–21
  aggregate societal costs, 15–16
  caregiver burden, 20
  direct and indirect costs, 14–16
  medication-assisted treatment, 16–17
  treatment costs, 14, 16–17
  unaccounted costs, 20–21
  underestimated costs, 18–19
  urine drug testing, 17–18
  workplace/productivity costs, 19–20
Council of Economic Advisors, 18–19
CPP. *See* condition place preference
creams, cannabis, 121
CRPS. *See* complex regional pain syndrome
CSA. *See* Controlled Substances Act
current opioid misuse measure (COMM), 159

dabbing, 111
DDS. *See* Descriptor Differential Scale
DEA. *See* Drug Enforcement Administration
delta opioid receptors (DORs), 183
depression, and chronic pain, 141
Descriptor Differential Scale (DDS), 168
detoxification, opioid, 17, 34, 162. *See also* withdrawal, opioid
Devane, William, 57
Diagnostic and Statistical Manual of Mental Disorder, Fifth Edition (*DSM-5*), 23, 24, 133
  definition of OUD, 25–27
diclofenac, 202
dispensaries, medical marijuana, 108
DORs. *See* delta opioid receptors
dosage of opioids, 157, 160–161, 227–228
DOSE. *See* Dronabinol Opioid Sparing Evaluation
Dravet syndrome, 95
driving, and cannabis use, 131
dronabinol, 83, 169, 196
  capsules (Marinol®), 89–90
  oral solution (Syndros®), 92–93
Dronabinol Opioid Sparing Evaluation (DOSE), 204
drug classifications in United States, 46

Drug Enforcement Administration (DEA), 33, 45, 48
DSM-5. See Diagnostic and Statistical Manual of Mental Disorder, Fifth Edition
dysmenorrhea, 148

ECS. *See* endocannabinoid system
edibles, cannabis, 116, 118–119, 126
emotional distress, 29
employment termination, and cannabis use, 51–52
endocannabinoid system (ECS), 61, 116, 167, 170, 171, 180–181, 183
   brain functions affected by, 57–58
   definition of, 179
   discovery of, 55–59
   endocannabinoids, 59, 61, 63–64
   evolution of, 59–60
   and medical school curriculum, 60–61
   opioid sparing medications that work via, 207
   receptors, 59, 63, 64–66
      effect, 61
      interaction of cannabinoids with, 66
   regulatory functions of, 60
   retrograde inhibition, 67
   treatments, health benefits of, 62–63
endogenous opioid peptides, 180
endorphins, 27
entourage effect, 83
extended-release/long-acting opioids, 155

FAAH. *See* fatty acid amidohydrolase
farm bill (2018), 47, 102
Farr, Sam, 49
fatty acid amidohydrolase (FAAH), 205
FDA. *See* Food and Drug Administration
fentanyl, 8, 152
fibromyalgia (FM), 142–143, 167, 169, 170

First Amendment, 50
flower, cannabis, 109–110
FM. *See* fibromyalgia
Food and Drug Administration (FDA), 10, 48, 74, 83, 85, 102, 192
   cannabinoid medications approved by, 87–88, 89–93, 95–100, 101
   medications approved for use in MAT by, 16–17
Frank, Barney, 47
functional gastrointestinal disorders, 148

gabapentin, 201, 203–204
Gaoni, Yehiel, 55
geraniol, 80
Guidelines for Prescribing Opioids for Chronic Pain (CDC), 4, 157, 213–214

H2. *See* Histamine-2
Hanus, Lumir, 57
headache. *See* chronic daily headache (CDH)
health effects of cannabis abuse, 131–133
heart rate, and cannabis use, 128
hemp, 40, 44, 47–48, 74, 76, 102, 195. *See also* cannabis
heroin, 8, 28, 29, 188
high-impact chronic pain, 140
Hinchey, Maurice, 49
Histamine-2 (H2), 60
HIV-associated cachexia, 89, 91, 93
HIV-associated neuropathic pain, 168
Howlett, Allyn, 57
hydrocodone, 152

IASP. *See* International Association for the Study of Pain
IBD. *See* inflammatory bowel disease
IBS. *See* irritable bowel syndrome
ICD-11. See *International Classification of Diseases*

immediate-release/short-acting opioids, 154–155, 157, 160
immune system, and chronic pain, 141
industrial hemp, 40, 44, 47, 74
Industrial Hemp Farming Act, 47
inflammatory bowel disease (IBD), 76
inflammatory pain, 141, 167, 170, 193
Institute of Medicine (IOM), 153
International Association for the Study of Pain (IASP), 3–4
International Classification of Diseases (ICD-11), 142
IOM. *See* Institute of Medicine
irritable bowel syndrome (IBS), 148
isolate cannabinoid medications
  cannabidiol (Epidiolex®), 95–98, 120
  contraindications of, 100–101
  effectiveness of, 101
  nabiximols (Sativex®), 98–100, 121
Israel, medical marijuana program in, 60

JCAHO. *See* Joint Commission on Accreditation of Healthcare Organizations
Joint Commission on Accreditation of Healthcare Organizations (JCAHO), 152

kapa opioid receptors (KOR), 183
ketamine, 201, 203
KORs. *See* kapa opioid receptors

LBP. *See* lower back pain
Lennox–Gastaut syndrome, 96, 97
lidocaine, 204
limonene, 80, 81
linalool, 80, 82
lower back pain (LBP), 139, 142, 144–145

Marihuana Tax Act (1937), 44
marijuana. *See* cannabis

marijuana use disorder, 133
MAT. *See* medication-assisted treatment
McPartland, John, 59
Mechoulam, Raphael, 55, 57
MED. *See* Morphine Equivalent Dose
medical marijuana, 10, 205. *See also* cannabis
  approved ailments, 47
  edibles, 116, 118–119
  healthcare provider recommendations, 50–51
  laws, states with, 45
  legal considerations for patients, 51–52
  and opioid use disorder, 186
  oral mucosal tinctures/extracts, 120–121
  preparations, CBD:THC ratio of, 196
  programs, 60, 107–108
  role of dispensaries, 108
  smoking, 113–114, 115
  as substitute for opioids, 194–195
  suppositories, 121–122
  topicals, 121
  vaporization, 114, 115–116
medication-assisted treatment (MAT), 10, 14, 32
  costs, 16–17
  and relapse rates, 187
mental effects of cannabis use, 130
Mental Health Parity and Addiction Equity Act (MHPAEA), 14
menthol, 204
meperidine, 152
methadone, 10, 16, 32, 33, 152, 158, 161, 185
MHPAEA. *See* Mental Health Parity and Addiction Equity Act
migraine headaches, 147
mood disorders, 29, 30
morphine, 157, 183, 186, 193, 206
Morphine Equivalent Dose (MED), 199–200
MORs. *See* mu-opioid receptors

motivation, 27–29
MS. *See* multiple sclerosis
mu-opioid receptors (MORs), 27, 31, 181
　allosteric modulation of, 183, 193
　and interaction with cannabinoid receptors, 183–184
multiple sclerosis (MS), 169, 170, 194, 196
muscle relaxants, 10
musculoskeletal pain, chronic, 148
mycrene, 80, 81

N-methyl-d-aspartate (NMDA) receptor, 49, 203
nabilone (Cesamet®) capsules, 90–92
nabiximols (Sativex®), 98–100, 101, 121, 169, 171, 194, 196
naloxone, 17, 33, 158, 161
naltrexone, 16, 34
Narcotics Anonymous, 33
National Academies of Sciences, Engineering, and Medicine, 166
National Institute on Drug Abuse (NIDA), 26, 48, 126, 127
　Modified ASSIST form, 26, 217–225
　Quick Screen, 215–216
　simplified screening for opioid use disorder, 26–27
National Poison Data System, 132
nausea, and cannabis use, 129
negative reinforcement, and opioid withdrawal, 27
neonatal abstinence syndrome, 19
nerolidol, 83
neuroadaptation, and opioids, 28
neuropathic pain, 140
　cannabinoid medications for, 167–168, 169, 205
　chronic, 146
　gabapentin for, 203–204
　HIV-associated, 168
　opioids for, 201
NIDA. *See* National Institute on Drug Abuse

NMDA. *See* N-methyl-d-aspartate receptor
nociceptive pain, 140
nonsteroidal antiinflammatory drugs (NSAIDs), 8, 202, 204, 205
NRS. *See* Numerical Rating Scale
NSAIDs. *See* nonsteroidal antiinflammatory drugs
Numerical Rating Scale (NRS), 168

ocimene, 81
Ogden Memo (2009), 48
OIC. *See* opioid-induced constipation
oil cartridge vapor pens, 116, 117
opioid epidemic, 5
　associated consequences of, 5
　costs. *See* costs of opioid epidemic
　dependency and abuse, 8
　national opioid overdose deaths, 9
　response to, 8, 10
opioid-induced constipation (OIC), 20–21, 159
opioid-induced hyperalgesia, 153
opioid sparing, 8, 10, 186, 191, 194, 199–200
　for acute pain, 201
　benefits of, 200
　cannabinoid medications for, 205–206
　　studies, 206
　for chronic pain, 201–202
　medications, 207
　traditional, 202–204
opioid use disorder (OUD), 8, 18, 158, 161, 162, 183, 186
　co-occurring psychiatric conditions, 29–30
　complications of, 24
　costs of. *See* costs of opioid epidemic
　definition of, 23–24
　DSM-5 definition of, 25–27
　early remission of, 25
　environmental influences, 31

opioid use disorder (OUD) (cont.)
  epidemiology of, 30
  medically supervised withdrawal, 34
  NIDA simplified screening for, 26–27
  overdose reversal, 33–34
  and pharmacogenetics, 31–32
  reward and motivation, 27–29
  risk factors for, 30–31
  screening, 31
  severity of, 25
  sustained remission of, 26
  treatment of, 14, 17, 32–33, 187
opioid weaning, 187
opioidergic agent, 179
opioidergic system, 179
opioids, 5, 27, 180
  adverse effects of, 20
  benefits from, 6–7
  for chronic pain, 201
    discontinuation, 158, 161–162
    duration and follow-up, 157–158, 160–161
    initiation and continuation, 157
    noncancer chronic pain, current guidelines, 153
    risk assessment and addressing harms, 159–160
    scientific evidence, 154
  combination with cannabinoid medications. See under cannabinoid medications (CMs)
  combination with other drugs, 156, 157, 161, 195
  dependence, 161
  dosage, 157–158, 160–161
  extended-release/long-acting, 155
  immediate-release/short-acting, 154–155, 157
  intoxication, signs and symptoms of, 25
  long-term effects of, 6
  Morphine Equivalent Dose of, 199–200
  and MORs, 181
  vs. nonopioid medications, 7
  overdose. See under overdose, drug
  treatment agreement, 160
  treatment considerations, 156
    CDC, 157–158
  types of, 154–156
  use, history of, 151–152
oral mucosal tinctures/extracts, cannabis, 120–121
OUD. See opioid use disorder
overdose, drug
  deaths, 8, 9, 18, 19, 56
  dronabinol, 90
  nabilone, 92
  nabiximols, 100
  opioids, 5, 6, 24, 33, 158, 160
    deaths, 8, 9, 18, 19, 181, 182
    signs and symptoms of, 34
  unintentional cannabis overdose, 132
oxycodone, 152, 202

pain, 3, 4. See also chronic pain
  classification of, 140–141
  definition of, 3–4
  as fifth vital sign, 152–153
  recent issues in, 4
pain medication questionnaire (PMQ), 159
palmitoylethanolamide (PEA), 195
para-aminophenol, 207
patches, cannabis, 121
patents for cannabis/cannabis-related inventions, 49
Paul, Ron, 47
PDMP. See prescription drug monitoring program
PEA. See palmitoylethanolamide
phantom limb pain, 145
pharmacogenetics, and opioid use disorder, 31–32
physical effects of cannabis use, 127
  breathing problems, 127–128
  child development problems during/after pregnancy, 128–129
  heart rate, increased, 128
  intense nausea and vomiting, 129
  stroke, 129

PMQ. *See* pain medication questionnaire
positive reinforcement, 27
posttraumatic stress disorder (PTSD), 29, 61
pregabalin, 201, 203–204
pregnancy
  and cannabinoid medications, 101
  child development problems during/after, 128–129
  opioid use/misuse during, 19, 32
prescription drug monitoring program (PDMP), 158, 159
presenteeism, 17, 19, 20
primary pain syndromes, 142
  complex regional pain syndrome, 143–144
  fibromyalgia, 142–143
  nonspecific lower back pain, 144–145
productivity costs of opioid epidemic, 19–20
PTSD. *See* posttraumatic stress disorder

qualitative urine drug testing, 17–18
quantitative urine drug testing, 17–18

reflex sympathetic dystrophy. *See* complex regional pain syndrome (CRPS)
rehabilitation, drug, 14, 17, 18, 29
relapse, opioid, 10, 33, 187–188
retrograde inhibition, by endocannabinoids, 67
reward system, 27–29
rimonabant, 88
ROF. *See* rofecoxib
rofecoxib (ROF), 202
Rohrabacher, Dana, 49
Rohrabacher–Farr Amendment (2014), 49–50
roll-ons, cannabis, 121

salves, cannabis, 121
Schedule 1 drugs, 45, 46, 102
Schedule 2 drugs, 46, 90, 92
Schedule 3 drugs, 46, 90
Schedule 4 drugs, 46
Schedule 5 drugs, 96
screener and opioid assessment for patients with pain (SOAPP), 159
secondary pain syndromes, 142
  chronic cancer-related pain, 145
  chronic daily headache, 147
  chronic musculoskeletal pain, 148
  chronic neuropathic pain, 146
  chronic postsurgical/posttraumatic pain, 145
  chronic visceral pain, 147–148
serotonin, 60
shatter, 110, 111, 112
Shen-Nung, 43
side effects of cannabis use, 125–126
  factors that affect reaction to cannabis, 125–126
  long-term, 127
  mental effects, 130
  physical effects, 127–130
  short-term, 126
single molecule drugs, vs. botanical drugs, 85
smoking, cannabis, 113–114, 115
  and breathing problems, 127–128
  and heart rate, 128
  oral health effects, 130
SOAPP. *See* screener and opioid assessment for patients with pain
somatosensory system, 140, 146
spasms, 170–171, 194
spasticity, 169, 170–171, 194
stroke, and cannabis use, 129
substance use disorders (SUDs), 23, 25. *See also* opioid use disorder (OUD)
SUDs. *See* substance use disorders
SUPPORT for Patients and Communities Act (2018), 16
suppositories, cannabis, 122–123
swelling, 167, 170

synthetic cannabinoid medications, 88
  contraindications of, 88–89
  dronabinol capsules (Marinol®), 89–90
  dronabinol oral solution (Syndros®), 92–93
  nabilone capsules (Cesamet®), 90–92

Tashkin, Donald, 113
terpenes, 80–83. *See also* cannabinoids
  binding to receptors, 66
  chart, 81–83
  entourage effect, 83
  odor of, 80
terpineol, 80
terpinolene, 82
delta-9-tetrahydrocannabinol (THC), 40, 42, 51, 55, 57, 73–74, 77, 80, 83, 92, 98–99, 100, 111, 116, 121, 126, 167, 168, 169, 170, 171, 172, 183, 186, 205
  binding to receptors, 66
  CBD:THC ratio, 84, 172
  -induced driving-performance, 131
  mental effects of, 130
  molecular structure of, 58, 74
  properties of, 74
tetrahydrocannabivarin (THCV), 78
THC. *See* delta-9-tetrahydrocannabinol
THCV. *See* tetrahydrocannabivarin
tolerance, opioid, 27, 29, 183, 185, 186, 191
topicals
  analgesics, 207
  cannabis, 121
  NSAIDs, 204

treatment costs of opioid epidemic, 14, 16–17
TRPV1 receptor. *See* capsaicin receptor
12-step program, 16, 17
21st Century Act, 16

UDT. *See* urine drug testing
unintentional cannabis overdose, 132
University of Mississippi School of Pharmacy, National Center for Natural Products Research, 48
urine drug testing (UDT), 8, 158, 159
  costs, 17–18
US Department of Health and Human Services, 50
US Department of Justice, 48–49, 50
US Patent and Trademark Office, 49

vaporization, cannabis, 114, 116
vaporizers, types of, 115, 116
visceral pain, chronic, 147–148
vital signs, 152
vomiting, and cannabis use, 129

water pipes, 114, 115
WHO. *See* World Health Organization
whole plant extracts, cannabinoid medications, 101
Wilkinson Memo (2014), 49
withdrawal, opioid, 27–28, 32, 161, 187
  and cannabinoid medications, 184, 185, 187, 191–192
  medically supervised, 34
  symptoms, 28, 161
workplace costs of opioid epidemic, 19–20
World Health Organization (WHO), 3